T0122195

Computer-Aided Analysis of Gastrointestinal Videos

Jorge Bernal · Aymeric Histace
Editors

Computer-Aided Analysis of Gastrointestinal Videos

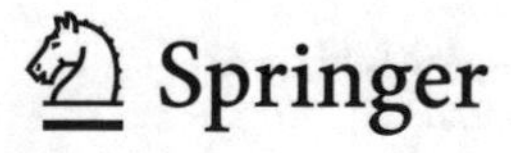

Editors
Jorge Bernal
Computer Vision Center and Computer
Science Department
Autonomous University of Barcelona
Bellaterra, Barcelona, Spain

Aymeric Histace
ETIS UMR 8051 (CY Paris Cergy
University, ENSEA, CNRS)
École Nationale Supérieure de
l'Electronique et de ses Applications
Cergy, France

ISBN 978-3-030-64342-3 ISBN 978-3-030-64340-9 (eBook)
https://doi.org/10.1007/978-3-030-64340-9

This Springer imprint is published by the registered company Springer Nature Switzerland AG
The registered company address is: Gewerbestrasse 11, 6330 Cham, Switzerland

Dedicated to the late Arnau Real: good student, great fellow and awesome human-being and friend. Your memories will be forever in our hearts.

Foreword

It is my great pleasure to see the publication of Gastrointestinal Image Analysis edited by Prof. Jorge Bernal del Nozal and Prof. Aymeric Histace. They are a pioneer and a central figure of the research field of computer-aided detection/diagnosis of colorectal polyps, an area I have been working in as well. This world's first, unique book gathers amazing results obtained from the Gastrointestinal Image ANAalysis (GIANA) challenge 2017 and 2018 (an official project endorsed by the MICCAI society), in which participants submitted detection, segmentation, or classification algorithms for colonoscopy or Wireless Capsule Endoscopy (WCE) videos for competition. I believe this ambitious challenge will definitely contribute to acceleration of the research on Artificial Intelligence (AI) for gastrointestinal endoscopy, ultimately resulting in improvement of quality of endoscopy which is yet to be standardized at all in "real" clinical practice; the Adenoma Detection Rate (ADR), the most important quality indicator for colonoscopy, varies according to endoscopists' expertise, strongly affecting the incidence of post-colonoscopy CRC and related mortality [3, 4]. I think this issue of the ADR would be one of the largest problems that gastrointestinal endoscopy practice harbours.

To change this unfavourable situation, researchers devoted to computer vision have been trying to adopt AI technologies. As the data described in this book show, the performance of AI for polyp detection/segmentation has surprisingly improved in comparison with the previous reports probably because of the application of advanced deep learning technologies and the improvement of hand-crafted feature extraction. Given the AI tools have potential to evolve the quality of colonoscopy regardless of the endoscopists' skill, they will have greater benefits for patient care than we expected. However, at the same time, we should bear in mind that the results of experimental studies are not always translated to clinical practice; there is a wide gap between ex vivo and in vivo studies [5].

To overcome this critical hurdle, we, clinical researchers, should assess the AI's potential in practical settings where the AI tools will be used in a real-time fashion during colonoscopy. Unfortunately, the number of such prospective studies is very limited; however, it is expected to increase because clinical researchers in this area are now shifting their focus to prospective evaluation. Ultimately, these AI tools should be validated in trials with long-term follow-up, and CRC incidence and mortality as the main outcome measures.

I believe this book will be an indispensable guide not only for engineers/researchers working on computer vision but also clinicians who are keen on future perspective of colonoscopy and WCE practice. I sincerely hope it will find the widest readership it doubtlessly deserves.

Yuichi Mori
Digestive Disease Center
Showa University Northern Yokohama Hospital
Yokohama, Kanagawa, Japan

Acknowledgements

- Aymeric Histace, Xavier Dray, Romain Leenhardt acknowledge CY Initiative for their finanical support through the « SmartVideoclonocopy » grant, ERGANEO for their financial support through grant 184 « Ipolyp ».
- Jorge Bernal and Aymeric Histace want to acknowledge « Société Française d'Endoscopie Digestive » for their financial support that made it possible to reward winners of GIANA17 and 18 challenges.
- **CVC-UAB**: This work was supported by the Spanish Government through the funded project HISINVIA (PI17/00894), by the Secretaria d'Universitats i Recerca de la Generalitat de Catalunya (SGR-2017-1669) and by CERCA Programme/Generalitat de Catalunya.
- **Hospital Clinic**: This work was supported by the Spanish Government through the funded project HISINVIA (PI17/00894), by the Foundation of the Spanish Society of Digestive Endoscopy (FSEED) and by the Secretaria d'Universitats i Recerca de la Generalitat de Catalunya (SGR-2017-653).
- **UMinho**: This work is supported by FCT (Fundação para a Ciência e Tecnologia) with the reference Project UID/EEA/04436/2019 and with the Ph.D. Grant SFRH/BD/92143/2013.
- **LIP6**: Thanks to Institut Universitaire d'ingénierie en Sante(IUIS) for supporting the works during the thesis of Orlando Chuquimia.
- **SFU**: Saeed Izadi and Ghassan Hamarneh acknowledge funding from the Natural Sciences and Engineering Research Council (NSERC) of Canada through the Collaborative Health Research Projects (CHRP), and NVIDIA Corporation for the donation of a Titan X GPU used in this research.
- **UCLAN**: Bogdan J. Matuszewski's contributions to the manuscript were in part supported by the Science and Technology Facilities Council (STFC) Cancer Diagnosis Network+ (CDN+).
- **NTNU**: IQ-MED: Image Quality enhancement in MEDical diagnosis, monitoring and treatment, project no. 247689.
- **Neuromation**: The work of Sergey Nikolenko was supported by the Russian Basic Research Foundation grant RFBR 18-54-74005 $EMBL\_t$.

- **UB**: This work was supported by the Spanish Government through the funded project RTI2018-095232-B-C21, by the Secretaria d'Universitats i Recerca de la Generalitat de Catalunya (SGR-2017-172).
- **MIRC**: Tom Eelbode and Raf Bisschops are supported by a grant of the Research Foundation Flanders (FWO). Frederik Maes is supported by Internal Funds KU Leuven under grant number C24/18/047 and by funding from the Flemish Government (AI Research Program).
- **CUENDO**: The work was supported in part by Hong Kong General Research Fund and Hong Kong Innovation and Technology Fund.

Introduction

This book presents the first comprehensive analysis of Gastrointestinal Image Analysis systems. These systems aim to assist clinicians in several critical clinical tasks such as are lesion detection in colonoscopy images or lesion classification in wireless capsule endoscopy imaging.

When writing this book, several objectives were identified. First of all, we wanted to focus on those clinical tasks that have been identified by clinicians as critical. Second, we wanted to take the chance to fully present the different methodologies that have concurred in the two iterations of GIANA challenge which is organized by the editors of this book. Going beyond a simple journal paper allows us to give the different teams to explain their methodologies with the depth they wanted. Third, as we are worried not only by the development but also by the validation of our methodologies, we wanted to fully introduce the different validation frameworks that we have used in the challenge and that will be available to anyone interested to do research in the topic.

We have designed the structure of the book with these objectives in mind, being its content divided into four different parts. The Part I deals with the clinical and technical context of the different target tasks that will be targeted. We present an overview of the clinical drawbacks that current clinical practice present and we explore which technical challenges should be faced in order to provide expected performance levels.

The Part II of the book is devoted to the explanation of the different methodologies that will be validated in this book. Each of the teams has a different chapter in which to explain their approach to solve the different tasks that are targeted. For those using deep learning approaches a similar structure has been proposed: the main architecture is introduced and then modifications over this baseline are presented in depth.

The Part III of the book deals with the explanation of the three different validation frameworks for polyp detection, polyp segmentation and wireless capsule endoscopy lesion analysis. We introduce each of the datasets and we present the different performance metrics that will be used to compare methods performance.

The Part IV of the book presents and analyzes the results of the different teams that concurred to GIANA 2017 and 2018 challenges. For the case of those tasks that were exactly the same in both iterations, we made an additional study aiming to observe if there were an evolution in the performance achieved by the best methodology and, for the case of the teams that concurred in both editions, we observe if there were significant changes in method performance.

We hope we have been able to fulfill our objectives and that this book offers a pleasant reading.

Jorge Bernal
Aymeric Histace

Contents

Part I Clinical Context

1 **Clinical Context for Intelligent Systems in Colonoscopy** 3
Gloria Fernández-Esparrach and Ana García-Rodríguez

2 **Clinical Context for Wireless Capsule Endoscopy Image Analysis** 9
Romain Leenhardt, Xavier Dray, and Aymeric Histace

Part II Technical Context

3 **Technical Context for Intelligent Systems in Colonoscopy** 17
F. Javier Sánchez, Yael Tudela, Marina Riera, and Jorge Bernal

4 **Technical Context for Wireless Capsule Endoscopy Image Analysis** 33
Aymeric Histace

Part III Methodologies

5 **Combination of Color-Based Segmentation, Markov Random Fields and Multilayer Perceptron** 41
Pedro Miguel Vieira, Nuno Renato Freitas, Carla Rolanda, and Carlos Santo Lima

6 **Hand Crafted Method: ROI Selection and Texture Description** 49
Orlando Chuquimia, Bertrand Granado, Xavier Dray, and Andrea Pinna

7 **AECNN: Adversarial and Enhanced Convolutional Neural Networks** 59
Saeed Izadi and Ghassan Hamarneh

8 **Dilated ResFCN and SE-Unet for Polyp Segmentation** 63
Yunbo Guo and Bogdan J. Matuszewski

9 **Multi-encoder Decoder Network for Polyp Detection** 75
Ahmed Mohammed and Marius Pedersen

10 **Multi-resolution Multi-task Network and Polyp Tracking** 81
Hanbo Chen

11 **Region-Based Convolutional Neural Network for Polyp Detection and Segmentation** 91
Hemin Ali Qadir, Ilangko Balasingham, and Younghak Shin

12 **ResNet** 99
Isabel Amaya-Rodriguez, Isabel Amaya-Rodriguez, Javier Civit-Masot, Francisco Luna-Perejon, Lourdes Duran-Lopez, Alexander Rakhlin, Sergey Nikolenko, Satoshi Kondo, Pablo Laiz, Jordi Vitrià, Santi Seguí, and Patrick Brandao

13 **Multi-scale Ensemble of ResNet Variants** 115
Joost van der Putten and Farhad Ghazvinian Zanjani

14 **Convolutional LSTM** 121
Tom Eelbode, Pieter Sinonquel, Raf Bisschops, and Frederik Maes

15 **TernausNet** 127
Vladimir I. Iglovikov and Alexey A. Shvets

16 **Regression-Based Convolutional Neural Network with a Tracker** 133
Ruikai Zhang and Carmen C. Y. Poon

17 **Other Methodologies** 141
Jorge Bernal and Aymeric Histace

Part IV Experimental Setup

18 **Polyp Detection in Colonoscopy Videos** 147
Jorge Bernal, Gloria Fernández, Ana García-Rodríguez, Yael Tudela, Marina Riera, and F. Javier Sánchez

19 **Polyp Segmentation in Colonoscopy Images** 151
Jorge Bernal, Gloria Fernández, Ana García-Rodríguez, and F. Javier Sánchez

20 **Wireless Capsule Endoscopy Image Analysis** 155
Aymeric Histace, Romain Leenhardt, and Xavier Dray

Part V Experimental Results and Analysis

21 **Polyp Detection in Colonoscopy Videos** 163
Jorge Bernal, Yael Tudela, Marina Riera, and F. Javier Sánchez

22 Polyp Segmentation in Colonoscopy Images 171
Jorge Bernal and Arnau Real

23 Wireless Capsule Endoscopy Image Analysis 177
Aymeric Histace

24 Conclusions and Perspectives 183
Jorge Bernal and Aymeric Histace

List of Figures

Fig. 1.1 Pie charts present the distribution of cases and deaths for the 10 most common cancers in 2018 for both sexes. *Source* GLOBOCAN 2018: overall, colorectal cancer ranks third in terms of incidence but second in terms of mortality 4
Fig. 2.1 Images and diagram showing the composition of a video capsule endoscope. References: Royal Free Hospital - London/UK 10
Fig. 2.2 Illustration of (left) PillCamSB3 and (right) Capsovision WCE with a lateral sensors for non-conventional image acquisition of the small intestine. Respectively taken from VideoDigest2017 and www.ortoday.com 12
Fig. 3.1 Image showing a complete endoluminal scene with several elements on it 26
Fig. 4.1 Intestines morphology 34
Fig. 4.2 Some examples of WCE images presenting with GIA 35
Fig. 4.3 Some examples of WCE images presenting with IBL 35
Fig. 5.1 Neighborhood system of 8 pixels used 44
Fig. 5.2 Two examples of results with training images. **a** Original image. **b** Component a from CIELab. **c** Component a from CIELab after pre-processing step. **d** Segmentation result 46
Fig. 6.1 Proposed system scheme of polyps detection 50
Fig. 6.2 Convolutional kernel model 51
Fig. 6.3 The Googlenet CNN 52
Fig. 6.4 Input image and the output of convolutional kernel number 13 52
Fig. 6.5 **a** Block matching with 1 neighborhood. **b** Block matching with 2 neighborhoods. **c** ROI validated in the image I_{n-1}. **d** 8 candidate motion vectors. **e** 8 candidate blocks displaced by the candidate motion vectors. **f** Candidate block having the lowest intensity standard variation SAD_{ij} ... 54

Fig. 6.6 Example of results obtained with the proposed methodology 57
Fig. 7.1 The schematic of the proposed AECNN model for polyp segmentation. The error in the discriminator is backpropagated through the segmenter to make it produce more realistic segmentation masks 60
Fig. 8.1 The structure of FCN8s, FCN16s and FCN32s 66
Fig. 8.2 Regular convolution (**a**)–(**c**) and atrous convolution (**d**). **a** Regular convolution, with pooling stride 2 and 1 × 3 kernel. **b** Regular convolution, with pooling stride 1 and 1 × 3 kernel. **c** Regular convolution, with pooling stride 1 and 1 × 5 kernel. **d** Atrous convolution, with pooling stride 1, 1 × 5 kernel and dilation 2; kernel size is 5 but only 3 weights are trainable 66
Fig. 8.3 Dilated ResFCN polyp segmentation network, with the feature extraction sub-network (in blue) based on the ResNet, the multi-resolution classification sub-network (in yellow) based on the dilated convolution, and the fusion sub-network (in green) using bilinear interpolation 68
Fig. 8.4 SE-Unet polyp segmentation network with SE-module to introduce attention gating to better utilize information in the computed feature maps and atrous spatial pyramid pooling (ASPP) to effectively control receptive filed 69
Fig. 8.5 Visualization of the test-time data augmentation. The image on the left shows an input test image. Images in the middle represent rotated, in 15° intervals, versions of the original image; the corresponding results of the binary segmentation in the rotated image reference frame; and the results after restoration to the original image reference frame. The image on the right shows final segmentation results, superimposed on the original image, with (in red) and without (in blue) test-time augmentation 70
Fig. 8.6 Typical results obtained for the SD images using FCN8s, ResFCN, Dilated ResFCN and SE-Unet networks (Guo 2019). For each image: the left column shows the polyp occurrence confidence maps with the red colour representing the high confidence and blue colour representing the low confidence of a polyp presence; the right column shows the original images with superimposed red and blue contours representing the ground truth and segmentation results, respectively 71

Fig. 8.7 Number of polyps as a function of Dice index histograms obtained on validation data for different segmentation methods. The definition of the Dice index histogram bin intervals is given below the graph 72
Fig. 9.1 Multi-encoder decoder object segmentation network 76
Fig. 9.2 Y-Net: given an input image, it is fed to both encoders. The weights of the last convolution at each depth of the encoder are summed and concatenated to the same spatial depth of the decoder 77
Fig. 9.3 Visualization of different layers for Y-Net. Image on the left shows the early convolutions layer in the encoder block for the first convolution. Image on the right shows late-stage convolution layer at the decoder. It is evident from patterns that the proposed model is able to learn different appearance of polyp sizes and orientation 79
Fig. 10.1 Detailed architecture of multi-resolution multi-task supervised segmentation network 83
Fig. 10.2 Illustration of pipeline of polyp detection in endoscopic video stream 86
Fig. 10.3 Illustration of data pre-processing and training augmentation pipeline 87
Fig. 10.4 Six examples of prediction results by our proposed method. On the left side of each sub-figure shows the raw image overlapped with polyp center truth (white cross) and predicted polyp center (black cross). On the right side of each sub-figure is the comparison between predicted segmentation and the truth annotation overlaid on the dimmed raw image. White arrows pointing to potential polyps missed by human experts when annotating 88
Fig. 11.1 Faster R-CNN and Mask R-CNN architecture used for polyp detection and segmentation, respectively. They both share the same structure except there is an additional branch to predict mask in Mask R-CNN as highlighted in light blue 92
Fig. 11.2 A building block of residual network 93
Fig. 11.3 Inception module (Szegedy et al. 2015) 94
Fig. 11.4 Our proposed method for polyp detection. The Faster R-CNN provides RoIs to the FP reduction unit. The FP reduction unit classifies the RoIs as either TPs or FPs using temporal coherence information among a set of consecutive frames, and estimates the location of missed polyps using interpolation 95

Fig. 11.5 Our proposed method for polyp segmentation. The first Mask R-CNN is used as the main model and its output is always taken while the second Mask R-CNN is used as an auxiliary model to help detect missed polyps and refine the output masks 96
Fig. 11.6 A case which explains the benefit of our ensemble model 96
Fig. 12.1 Residual learning block 100
Fig. 12.2 ResNet-12 architecture 101
Fig. 12.3 Block diagram of the implemented approach 102
Fig. 12.4 ResNet-50 in faster convolutional neural network 103
Fig. 12.5 Block diagram of the implemented approach 103
Fig. 12.6 Processing applied to the original images. First, black edges are removed in a pre-processing step. Then data augmentation is applied, generating three different new images 104
Fig. 12.7 Neuromation architecture 106
Fig. 12.8 Basic network architecture 107
Fig. 12.9 Network architecture for WCE detection and localization task 108
Fig. 12.10 RTC-ATC Polyp detection results task. Left: polyps detected by Faster R-CNN. Confidence values are represented in blue. Right: their corresponding ground truth. A and B show the performance in case a polyp appears, while C shows the performance in case there is no polyp 110
Fig. 12.11 Neuromation results. Left to right: **a** original image, **b** ground truth, **c** predicted mask, **d** uncertainty of the prediction 112
Fig. 13.1 Schematic overview of the used models and the ensembling method. A given input image is fed to five different models with three different input resolutions. The outputs of the resulting 15 models are then finally fed to a small fully connected network to determine a final classification label 118
Fig. 14.1 Our proposed extension to Deeplabv3+ places a convLSTM layer after the high-level features are extracted. This gives the decoder network access to relevant semantic information from the previous frames 122

Fig. 15.1 These segmentation networks are based on encoder-decoder network of U-Net family. TernausNet uses pre-trained VGG16 network as an encoder, while AlbuNet34 uses pre-trained ResNet34 as an encoder. It is different from TernausNet in that it adds skip-connections to the upsampling path, while TernausNet concatenates downsampled layers with the upsampling path (just like original U-Net does). Each box corresponds to a multi-channel feature map. The number of channels is pointed below the box. The height of the box represents a feature map resolution. The blue arrows denote skip-connections where information is transmitted from the encoder to the decoder 128

Fig. 15.2 The prediction of our detector on the validation set image. Here, the left panel shows the original image, the middle panel shows the ground truth training mask, and the right panel shows the predicted mask. Green dots inside of each mask corresponds to the centroid that defines angiodysplasia localization output. Here, for example, the real and predicted values for centroid coordinates correspondingly are $p^1_{mask} = (376, 144)$, $p^1_{pred} = (380, 143)$ for the first mask and $p^2_{mask} = (437, 445)$, $p^2_{pred} = (437, 447)$ for the second mask 130

Fig. 16.1 Pipeline of the proposed computer-aided detection algorithm RYCO (Zhang et al. 2018) 134

Fig. 16.2 Residual learning module of our proposed ResYOLO detector 136

Fig. 16.3 Architecture of ResYOLO detector 138

Fig. 17.1 Proposed feature maps for exemplary angiodysplasia image patch 142

Fig. 18.1 Statistics of CVC-ClinicVideoDB database. PF stands for polyp frames, NPF for non-polyp frames, PC for Paris classification representing morphology of the polyp according (0-Is for sessile polyps, 0-Ip for pedunculated polyps and 0-IIa for flat-elevated polyps) and S for the size of the polyps (in mm) 148

Fig. 18.2 Example of the content of CVC-VideoClinicDB database. First pair of images shows a scene with a polyp and its corresponding binary ground truth mask, representing the polyp in the image. The second pair of images shows a scene without a polyp. In this case, ground truth is a black image 148

Fig. 18.3 List of participants in GIANA 2017 Challenge on the polyp detection and localization categories 149

Fig. 18.4 List of participants in GIANA 2018 Challenge on the polyp detection and localization categories 150
Fig. 19.1 Examples of content of SD segmentation training and testing datasets. The first two images show an original image and its corresponding ground truth from CVC-ColonDB whereas the last two ones show an original image from CVC-ClinicDB and its corresponding ground truth 152
Fig. 19.2 Examples of content of HD segmentation image dataset. Image on the left shows an original image showing a polyp whereas image on the right shows its associated binary mask annotation 152
Fig. 19.3 List of participants in GIANA 2017 Challenge on polyp segmentation (SD and HD categories) 153
Fig. 19.4 List of participants in GIANA 2018 Challenge on polyp segmentation (SD and HD categories) 154
Fig. 20.1 Some examples of WCE images extracted from the CAD-CAP database with related ground truth. First raw: Angiectasia, Second raw: Inflammatory lesions, Third raw: Normal images 157
Fig. 20.2 Confusion Matrix for GIANA 2018 158
Fig. 21.1 ROC curves for **a** polyp detection and **b** polyp localization from GIANA 2017 challenge 165
Fig. 21.2 ROC curves for **a** polyp detection and **b** polyp localization from GIANA 2018 challenge 168
Fig. 22.1 Example of some of the most challenging images for all teams regarding segmentation of SD images. Polyp regions are highlighted by a circle 173
Fig. 22.2 Example of some of the most challenging images for all teams regarding segmentation of HD images. Polyp regions are highlighted by a circle 174

List of Tables

Table 2.1 Technical comparisons of the existing WCE 11
Table 3.1 Summary of the main handcrafted methods 22
Table 3.2 Summary of the main approaches using machine learning 23
Table 3.3 Summary of polyp segmentation methods 25
Table 8.1 Mean Dice index obtained on 4-fold validation data using Dilated ResFCN network 71
Table 11.1 Augmentation strategies applied to enlarge the training dataset 97
Table 12.1 Polyps detection performance. TP: True Positive, FP: False Positive, TN: True Negative, FN: False Negative 110
Table 12.2 Results of classification task 112
Table 12.3 Results of localization task 112
Table 13.1 Base architecures used for this solution 117
Table 15.1 Segmentation results. Intersection over Union (IoU) and Dice coefficient (Dice) are in %, and inference time (Time) is in ms 131
Table 18.1 Performance metrics for polyp detection 149
Table 20.1 2017 Participating Team 159
Table 20.2 2018 Participating Team 159
Table 21.1 Polyp detection and localization results at GIANA 2017. Total number of images: 18103 (12592 with a polyp and 6141 without a polyp) 164
Table 21.2 Polyp detection and localization results at GIANA 2018. Total number of images: 18103 (12592 with a polyp and 6141 without a polyp) 166
Table 21.3 Summary of key results from the polyp detection task at GIANA 17 and 18 challenges 169
Table 21.4 Summary of key results from the polyp localization task at GIANA 17 and 18 challenges 169
Table 22.1 Polyp segmentation results. Total number of images: 612 SD images 172

Table 22.2 Polyp segmentation results. Total number of images: 150 HD images ... 174
Table 22.3 Summary of the most relevant polyp segmentation results in SD images over the two editions of the GIANA challenge. Total number of images: 612 SD images ... 175
Table 22.4 Summary of the most relevant polyp segmentation results in HD images over the two editions of the GIANA challenge. Total number of images: 150 HD images ... 175
Table 23.1 WCE angiodysplasia detection and localization results ... 178
Table 23.2 WCE lesion detection results ... 180
Table 23.3 WCE lesion localization results ... 180

Part I
Clinical Context

Chapter 1
Clinical Context for Intelligent Systems in Colonoscopy

Gloria Fernández-Esparrach and Ana García-Rodríguez

Colorectal cancer (CRC) is the third most common cancer in both sexes and the second leading cause of death in the world (Bray et al. 2018). Worldwide, 1.4 million new cases of CRC are diagnosed annually and the incidence rates are slightly higher in men than in women. The World Health Organization (WHO) reported a rate of mortality of 9.2% in 2018, as can be seen in Fig. 1.1.

CRC incidence rates vary widely. Incidence in developed countries tends to stabilize due to the implementation of screening programs, an issue that has been hampered in countries with limited resources (Favoriti et al. 2016). The disease can be considered a marker of socioeconomic development, with incidence rates that increase in parallel to the growth of developing countries, where people are adapting to western lifestyle (Arnold et al. 2017).

1.1 Risk Factors

Almost 90% of cases of CRC are sporadic, where an interaction between environmental factors and genetic susceptibility determines the onset and development of CRC. The diet probably influences colorectal carcinogenesis through the interaction of direct effects on the immune response and inflammation and the indirect effects of malnutrition and the risk of obesity for CRC. Calcium, fiber (whole grain) and milk have been associated with a lower risk of CRC whereas the intake of red and processed meat has been associated with an increased risk (Song et al. 2015). Tobacco

G. Fernández-Esparrach (✉) · A. García-Rodríguez
Endoscopy Unit, Gastroenterology Department, Hospital Clínic, ICMDiM,
University of Barcelona, Barcelona, Spain
e-mail: mgfernan@clinic.cat

IDIBAPS, CIBEREHD, Barcelona, Spain

J. Bernal and A. Histace (eds.), *Computer-Aided Analysis of Gastrointestinal Videos*,
https://doi.org/10.1007/978-3-030-64340-9_1

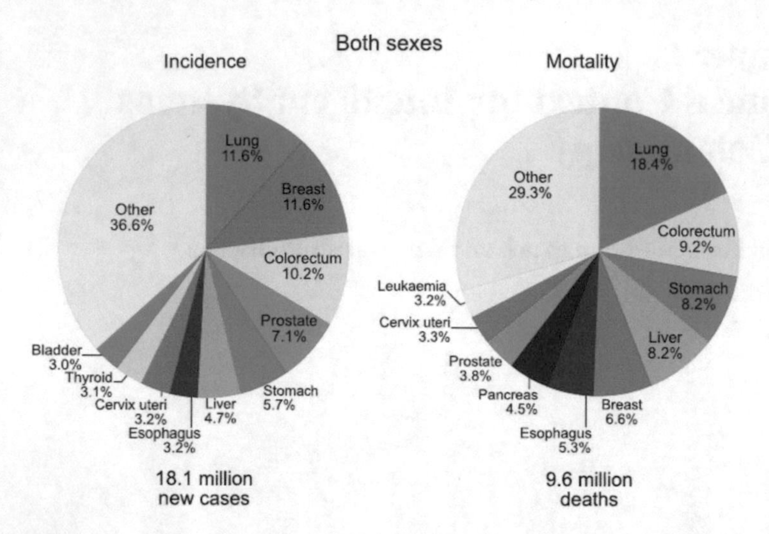

Fig. 1.1 Pie charts present the distribution of cases and deaths for the 10 most common cancers in 2018 for both sexes. *Source* GLOBOCAN 2018: overall, colorectal cancer ranks third in terms of incidence but second in terms of mortality

and alcohol consumption increase the risk of CRC too (Botteri et al. 2008; Cai et al. 2014). Modifications in diet and lifestyle are therefore an attractive strategy to reduce the overall burden of CRC.

1.2 Pathogenesis

CRC pathogenesis is due to the progressive accumulation of genetic and epigenetic alterations. Almost all CRC originate from a polyp, with an estimated progression time of 10–15 years, depending on the characteristics of the lesion and other independent risk factors (Kuipers et al. 2013).

From a histological point of view, polyps are classified as neoplastic and non-neoplastic, depending on whether or not they have a risk of degeneration. Neoplastic lesions include adenomas and serrated polyps. Neoplastic transformation affecting the colon epithelium is characterized by two distinct morphological pathways of carcinogenesis: the conventional adenoma-carcinoma sequence and the serrated pathway (Rex et al. 2012).

1.3 Management

Endoscopy is the most effective diagnostic and therapeutic tool for secondary and tertiary prevention of CRC, since it not only allows identification of polyps, but also allows removing them. On the other hand, optical advanced diagnosis can predict the histology of a polyp based on its endoscopic features.

Once identified, neoplastic polyps should be resected endoscopically in an en-bloc manner to allow a proper pathological diagnosis. Fortunately, most polyps are small in size (<10 mm) and have a low potential for malignancy (Lieberman et al. 2008). Therefore, the American Society for Gastrointestinal Endoscopy (ASGE) proposes "resect and discard" or "leave in situ" strategies for diminutive polyps (≤ 5 mm) of the colon and rectum and recto-sigma, respectively, to reduce the costs of histopathological analysis (Rex et al. 2011).

At present, the evidence is insufficient to secure benchmarks and extend the use of these strategies in daily clinical practice. Artificial Intelligence, through deep learning systems, emerges as a helpful tool to enable the recognition of polyps in real time (Mori et al. 2018). However, its effectiveness has not yet reached the sufficient level of performance in terms of applicability in clinical practice.

1.4 Current Limitations of White Light Endoscopy

Colonoscopy is not foolproof and still has some drawbacks. The reduced field of view of the optical camera placed at the tip of the endoscope ($<180°$), the polyp occultation produced by colon angulations and folds, the insufficient bowel preparation and the dependence on the experience of the endoscopist, result in a polyp miss rate of 22% and a risk of developing cancer after a negative colonoscopy of 8% (Van Rijn et al. 2006; Samadder et al. 2014). Currently, 12% of large adenomas (at least 1 cm) are missed even by expert endoscopists using meticulous techniques with the best available equipment, and these large adenomas are the ones that are most likely to transform into cancer. Factors such as quality of bowel cleansing and time spent examining the colonic mucosa have been shown to affect miss rates (Rex et al. 2015). For these reasons, several efforts have been made to improve the detection of polyps, which include better tolerated cleaning solutions, improvements in endoscopes, and accessory devices that increase mucosal visualization (Cheng et al. 2016; Bucci et al. 2014; Williet et al. 2018).

Nevertheless, the ambiguous in situ differential diagnosis of neoplastic from non-neoplastic polyps leads to an inefficient management and treatment of patients (delay in decision making, repetition of colonoscopies, and increased patient journey and risk) (Lee et al. 2014). This is because colonoscopy heavily relies on the subjective nonquantifiable visual assessments of colorectal polyps (e.g., polyp morphology and surface patterns), which is not considered sufficient evidence. For this reason, the "resect and discard" or "leave in situ" strategies for polyps <5 mm can only be used for experienced endoscopists with a reliable histological prediction capacity (Dayyeh et al. 2015).

In order to achieve a better histological prediction, several techniques have been developed. The most common technique is chromoendoscopy (with dyes or virtual). A meta-analysis published in 2015 (Dayyeh et al. 2015) including 20 studies that used Narrow Band Imagine (NBI), all in vivo and published between 2008 and 2014, showed that the pooled negative predictive value of NBI for adenomatous polyp histology was 91% (95% CI 88%, 94%).

During real-time optical diagnosis, validated optical diagnostic scales, such as the widely used NBI International Colorectal Endoscopic (NICE) classification should be used to improve diagnostic accuracy (Bisschops et al. 2019). No universal training system for differentiation between neoplastic and non-neoplastic colorectal polyps has been established yet. Several teaching modules, mostly computer-based, have been studied and some of them are showing promising results with respect to improving interobserver agreement; however, in a substantial number of studies the interobserver agreement was still moderate after training (Rastogi et al. 2014).

Considering the mentioned drawbacks of colonoscopy, three potential areas in which computer science may play a role have been identified:

1. Automatic polyp detection and localization: one of the drawbacks is related to the difficulty in detecting certain types of polyps such as small or flat lesions. Flat polyps can be detected with the support of CT (Fidler and Johnson 2009) although its detection supposes additional patient radiation and is limited by the size. Detection of small polyps cannot be undertaken with the help of CT as the current available resolution makes it impossible to detect polyps with size smaller than 10 mm, therefore the diagnosis in these cases should only rely on endoscopic exploration.
2. Polyp classification: the decision to perform polypectomy is commonly taken by an estimation of the size and histology of the detected lesion. This estimation is usually made by means of visual observation and therefore incorporates some degree of subjectivity. In this context, a system that can objectively provide an estimation of the size and classification of the polyp could allow taking in vivo diagnostic decisions and this would optimize the treatment timing.
3. Patients lesion follow-up and endoscopy navigation: there is a necessity expressed by some clinicians regarding the recognition of the area that a lesion occupies, which can be useful for two different reasons: (1) for the case of polyps that have not been removed, an univocal recognition of the lesion would allow the study of the evolution of the lesion; (2) an accurate recognition of the marks that clinicians leave to identify the area of the polyp once it is removed would allow the exploration of areas nearby the lesion to search for new pathologies.

References

Arnold, M., Sierra, M. S., Laversanne, M., Soerjomataram, I., Jemal, A., & Bray, F. (2017). Global patterns and trends in colorectal cancer incidence and mortality. *Gut*, *66*(4), 683–691.

Bisschops, R., East, J. E., Hassan, C., Hazewinkel, Y., Kamiński, M. F., Neumann, H., et al. (2019). Advanced imaging for detection and differentiation of colorectal neoplasia: European society of gastrointestinal endoscopy (ESGE) guideline–update 2019. *Endoscopy*, *51*(12), 1155–1179.

Botteri, E., Iodice, S., Bagnardi, V., Raimondi, S., Lowenfels, A. B., & Maisonneuve, P. (2008). Smoking and colorectal cancer: A meta-analysis. *The Journal of the American Medical Association*, *300*(23), 2765–2778.

Bray, F., Ferlay, J., Soerjomataram, I., Siegel, R. L., Torre, L., Jemal, A., et al. (2018). GLOBOCAN estimates of incidence and mortality worldwide for 36 cancers in 185 countries. *CA: A Cancer Journal for Clinicians*, *68*(6), 394–424.

Bucci, C., Rotondano, G., Hassan, C., Rea, M., Bianco, M. A., Cipolletta, L., et al. (2014). Optimal bowel cleansing for colonoscopy: Split the dose! a series of meta-analyses of controlled studies. *Gastrointestinal Endoscopy*, *80*(4), 566–576.

Cai, S., Li, Y., Ding, Y., Chen, K., & Jin, M. (2014). Alcohol drinking and the risk of colorectal cancer death: A meta-analysis. *European Journal of Cancer Prevention*, *23*(6), 532–539.

Cheng, J., Tao, K., Shuai, X., & Gao, J. (2016). Sodium phosphate versus polyethylene glycol for colonoscopy bowel preparation: An updated meta-analysis of randomized controlled trials. *Surgical Endoscopy*, *30*(9), 4033–4041.

Dayyeh, B. K. A., Thosani, N., Konda, V., Wallace, M. B., Rex, D. K., Chauhan, S. S., et al. (2015). ASGE technology committee systematic review and meta-analysis assessing the ASGE PIVI thresholds for adopting real-time endoscopic assessment of the histology of diminutive colorectal polyps. *Gastrointestinal Endoscopy*, *81*(3), 502–e1.

Favoriti, P., Carbone, G., Greco, M., Pirozzi, F., Pirozzi, R. E. M., & Corcione, F. (2016). Worldwide burden of colorectal cancer: A review. *Updates in Surgery*, *68*(1), 7–11.

Fidler, J., & Johnson, C. (2009). Flat polyps of the colon: Accuracy of detection by CT colonography and histologic significance. *Abdominal Imaging*, *34*(2), 157–171.

Kuipers, E. J., Rösch, T., & Bretthauer, M. (2013). Colorectal cancer screening-optimizing current strategies and new directions. *Nature Reviews Clinical Oncology*, *10*(3), 130.

Lee, T. J., Rees, C. J., Blanks, R. G., Moss, S. M., Nickerson, C., Wright, K. C., et al. (2014). Colonoscopic factors associated with adenoma detection in a national colorectal cancer screening program. *Endoscopy*, *46*(03), 203–211.

Lieberman, D., Moravec, M., Holub, J., Michaels, L., & Eisen, G. (2008). Polyp size and advanced histology in patients undergoing colonoscopy screening: Implications for CT colonography. *Gastroenterology, 135*(4), 1100–1105. https://doi.org/10.1053/j.gastro.2008.06.083.

Mori, Y., Kudo, S.-E., Misawa, M., Saito, Y., Ikematsu, H., Hotta, K., et al. (2018). Real-time use of artificial intelligence in identification of diminutive polyps during colonoscopy: A prospective study. *Annals of Internal Medicine*, *169*(6), 357–366.

Rastogi, A., Rao, D. S., Gupta, N., Grisolano, S. W., Buckles, D. C., Sidorenko, E., et al. (2014). Impact of a computer-based teaching module on characterization of diminutive colon polyps by using narrow-band imaging by non-experts in academic and community practice: A video-based study. *Gastrointestinal Endoscopy*, *79*(3), 390–398.

Rex, D. K., Kahi C, O'Brien, M., et al. (2011). The American society for gastrointestinal endoscopy PIVI (Preservation and Incorporation of Valuable Endoscopic Innovations) on real-time endoscopic assessment of the histology of diminutive colorectal polyps. *Gastrointest Endoscopy, 73*(3), 419–422. https://doi.org/10.1016/j.gie.2011.01.023.

Rex, D. K., Ahnen, D. J., Baron, J. A., Batts, K. P., Burke, C. A., Burt, R. W., et al. (2012). Serrated lesions of the colorectum: Review and recommendations from an expert panel. *The American Journal of Gastroenterology*, *107*(9), 1315.

Rex, D. K., Schoenfeld, P. S., Cohen, J., et al. (2015). Quality indicators for colonoscopy. *Gastrointest Endoscopy, 81*(1), 31–53. https://doi.org/10.1016/j.gie.2014.07.058.

Samadder, N. J., Curtin, K., Tuohy, T. M., Pappas, L., Boucher, K., Provenzale, D., et al. (2014). Characteristics of missed or interval colorectal cancer and patient survival: A population-based study. *Gastroenterology*, *146*(4), 950–960.

Song, M., Garrett, W. S., & Chan, A. T. (2015). Nutrients, foods, and colorectal cancer prevention. *Gastroenterology*, *148*(6), 1244–1260.

Van Rijn, J. C., Reitsma, J. B., Stoker, J., Bossuyt, P. M., Van Deventer, S. J., & Dekker, E. (2006). Polyp miss rate determined by tandem colonoscopy: A systematic review. *American Journal of Gastroenterology*, *101*(2), 343–350.

Williet, N., Tournier, Q., Vernet, C., Dumas, O., Rinaldi, L., Roblin, X., et al. (2018). Effect of Endocuff-assisted colonoscopy on adenoma detection rate: Meta-analysis of randomized controlled trials. *Endoscopy*, *50*(09), 846–860.

Chapter 2
Clinical Context for Wireless Capsule Endoscopy Image Analysis

Romain Leenhardt, Xavier Dray, and Aymeric Histace

2.1 Introduction

Wireless Capsule Endoscopy (WCE) takes the form of a pill equipped with a CCD or CMOS sensor, two batteries, and a RF (radiofrequency) transmitter, that enables the wireless identification of gastrointestinal abnormalities such as ulcers, blood, and polyps (Moglia et al. 2009) with no need for hospitalization or sedation.

Wireless Capsule Endoscopy (WCE) has rapidly become the standard minimally invasive method for visualization of the small bowel (SB). WCE is considered as the first-line investigation of SB diseases (Iddan et al. 2000) and may become the leading diagnostic tool for the entire gastrointestinal tract. With a mean number of 50,000 SB frames per video, SB-CE reading is time-consuming, tedious (30–40 min per video), and costly (McAlindon et al. 2016). This entails an inherent risk of missed lesions during the reading process by physicians.

In the last decade, WCE has become a breakthrough technology. Many fabricants such as Medtronics, IntroMedic, and Olympus (Gerber et al. 2007) have developed a variety of capsules for the complete examination of the gastrointestinal tract.

2.2 WCE Technical Aspects

Figure 2.1 shows the usual classic component layout of WCE.

A. Histace (✉)
ENSEA, ETIS UMR 8051 (CY Paris Cergy University, ENSEA, CNRS), 6 av. du Ponceau, 95014 Cergy, France
e-mail: aymeric.histace@ensea.fr

R. Leenhardt · X. Dray
APHP, Sorbonne Université, Paris, France

J. Bernal and A. Histace (eds.), *Computer-Aided Analysis of Gastrointestinal Videos*,
https://doi.org/10.1007/978-3-030-64340-9_2

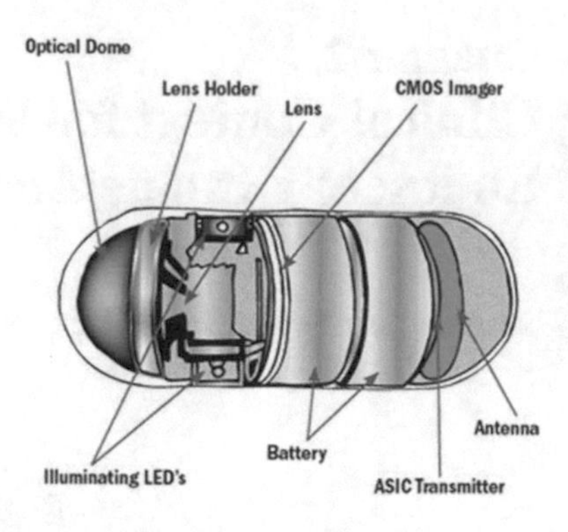

Fig. 2.1 Images and diagram showing the composition of a video capsule endoscope. References: Royal Free Hospital - London/UK

As it can be noticed, the battery is the element that occupies majority of available space in the capsule. The current autonomy is between 8 and 10 h by exam. Nevertheless, the average processing time from the mouth to the anus is more than 12 h, and, depending on the organism of the patient, sometimes even 24 h; under these conditions the capacity of this battery will be 55 mA @ 12 h, a very low one to supply enough power to the capsule. Currently the two batteries used in the WCE are composed of silver oxide, the only material approved for clinical use. Even if it is not the most efficiently solution, improvements are quite limited in this area: If others batteries were used, as lithium batteries that can provide longer operating times or carbon nanotubes that will produce at the same time a good autonomy while reducing the required space, the energy performance will be better. As an example, batteries composed of Zinc Air (ZnO2), will increase about four times the capacity and the weight will be reduced in 20%.

CMOS and CCD sensors are both used in WCE. The main characteristics of these technologies are as follows:

- CMOS (Complementary Oxide Silicone): A CMOS imager converts the charge to voltage within each pixel, using an array of pixels to convert light into electronic signals. This signal is weak and needs amplifying to a usable level, and then each pixel has its own amplifier circuit. The result is a lower chip count, an increased reliability, a reduced power consumption, and a more compact.
- CCD (Charge Coupled Device): The CCD imager transfers the charge from the pixel, created by photoelectric conversion, through a bucket relay transfer to the imager output stage. The charge transfer is almost complete, which means that noise is rare, but a high voltage differential is required to improve transfer efficiency, which increases power consumption.

The most recent WCE of Given Imaging company uses a CMOS sensor "Aptina MT9S526".

The transmission is one of the most important but consuming elements of the capsule, because it has to process about at least 150,000 images per exam (often more), this module is nearly 100%-active during the all exam. Currently, the capsules

Table 2.1 Technical comparisons of the existing WCE

	PillCam SB	EndoCapsule	MiroCam	Sayaka	OMOM	Vector
Size (mm)	26 × 11	26 × 11	24 × 11	23 × 9	28 × 13	26 × 11
Weight (gr)	3.7	3.8	3.3		6	
See angle	140	145	150	360	140	
LED	4	6	6	4	6	4
Rate (fps)	2	2	2–3	30	0.5, 1, 2	19
Image sensor	CMOS	CCD	CMOS		CCD	QVGA
Autonomy	8	8–10	9–11		8	5

could use either one of these systems for image transmission to the wearable data-logger:

- By RF-transmitter (Zarlink ZL70340 E3, for instance): composed of an oscillator and a control circuit that send images with a variable rate 800/400/200 kbps and a carrier frequency of 402–405 MHz, the nominal current is 5 and 1 mA in passive mode.
- By electric-field propagation: this system is a more experimental one used on the MIRO capsule. Based on a novel human telemetry technology known as electric-field propagation, it uses the human body as a conductive medium for data transmission. The transmitters are a pair of gold plates coated on the surface of the capsule, reducing drastically the power consumed compared with existing communication devices that use RF transmission technology. Thanks to a longer operation time, this capsule takes advantage of the surplus energy to produce more image data; the autonomy of this capsule is between 10 and 12 h but remains barely used by clinicians.

In Table 2.1, a comparison of the different existing technologies of WCE is proposed.

Very recent generations of videocapsules have strongly improved the quality of bowel investigation. PillCam SB3, for instance, compared to the previous SB2 generation showed a significant improvement in bleeding detection (Blanco-Velasco et al. 2019) but also on several other types of pathologies as largely reported in the literature. Increase of the image resolution, more important acquisition rate (up to 5 fps), non-conventional image sensors (see Fig. 2.2 and finally improved Graphical User Interface for physicians pave the way to strengthen the use of WCE for a broader field of applications).

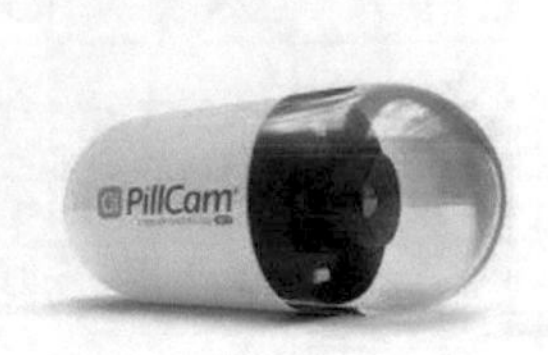

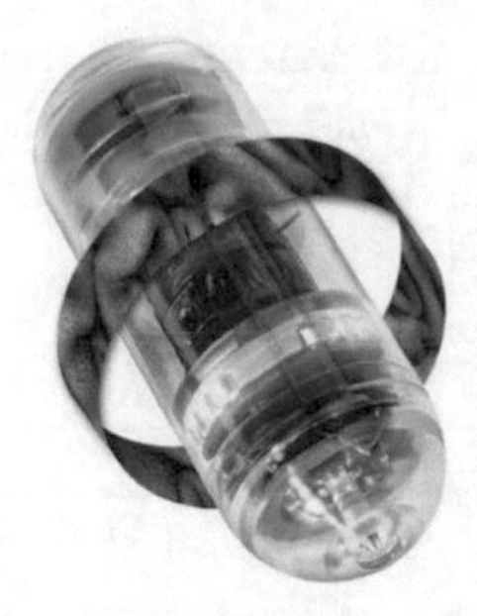

Fig. 2.2 Illustration of (left) PillCamSB3 and (right) Capsovision WCE with a lateral sensors for non-conventional image acquisition of the small intestine. Respectively taken from VideoDigest2017 and www.ortoday.com

2.3 Challenges in WCE

Current main issues of WCE are (Gerber et al. 2007):

- The complete analysis of the 150,000+ images is time-consuming for physicians, and even for experienced ones, WCE diagnoses are sometimes challenging.
- The transmission of the 150,000+ images, that represents 80% of the overall energy consumption of the embedded batteries, limits to 8 h the autonomy of the classic WCE, whereas 12 h are necessary to scan the complete intestinal tract.
- In the particular case of Colorectal Cancer, a recent study comparing diagnostic capabilities of videoendoscopy and of WCE shows that the average detection rate is around 80% polyps per patient (Spada et al. 2011; Eliakim et al. 2009). Thus, the improvement of polyp detection and classification capabilities of WCE is strongly expected from gastroenterologists.
- Processing capabilities of WCE are limited to transmit raw images. No "intelligence" is currently embedded into the imaging device itself.

Artificial intelligence (AI) has become the main focus in the last 10 years for Computer-aided analysis of the WCE images.

Nevertheless, AI-based solutions rely strongly on databases. Big data exploitation (epidemiology, predictive medicine) and signals analysis (EKG, EEG, imaging, pathology, dermatology, ophthalmology...) were the first successful application of AI in healthcare, followed by government approval. AI has a vast spectrum of potential applications in digestive endoscopy as well. AI can be used for screening, diagnosis, characterization, treatment, and prognosis evaluation, in a wide array of procedures. The quantity of published work in this field is thriving. Computer-assisted detection and characterization of colonic polyps, for instance, were amongst the first successful applications of AI and should be commercially available shortly. The automated reading of a capsule endoscopy is also very demonstrative of what AI will be able to accomplish in the next future.

It is believed that AI will significantly improve diagnostic performances and thus the quality of care. Today, endoscopists should not only promote this technological revolution, but also address new issues in the field of AI, regarding the respective roles of physicians (focused on ethics and patient-relations) and AI-machines (assistants vs autonomous), as well as responsibility (physicians vs. manufacturing companies), and reimbursement (physician vs manufacturing companies).

In Koulaouzidis et al. (2017), authors reported that incorporating machine learning algorithms into CE reading is difficult as large amounts of image annotations are required for training. They noted back that existing databases lack graphic annotations of pathologies and cannot be used for advancement of software solutions.

2.4 Conclusions

Based on this, it then appeared a real need for robust and reliable databases for WCE image analysis. GIANA challenge was the perfect opportunity to gather efforts and build a first database dedicated to WCE data and permitting the community to develop AI-based approaches that could be fairly compared in terms of performance.

References

Blanco-Velasco, G., Solórzano-Pineda, O., Mendoza-Segura, C., & Hernández-Mondragón, O. (2019). PillCam SB3 vs. PillCam SB2: Can technologic advances in capsule endoscopy improve diagnostic yield in patients with small bowel bleeding? *Revista de Gastroenterología de México (English Edition)*, *84*(4), 467–471.

Eliakim, R., Yassin, K., Niv, Y., Metzger, Y., Lachter, J., Gal, E., et al. (2009). Prospective multicenter performance evaluation of the second-generation colon capsule compared with colonoscopy. *Endoscopy*, *41*(12), 1026–1031.

Gerber, J., Bergwerk, A., & Fleischer, D. (2007). A capsule endoscopy guide for the practicing clinician: Technology and troubleshooting. *Gastrointestinal Endoscopy*, *66*(6), 1188–1195.

Iddan, G., Meron, G., Glukhovsky, A., & Swain, P. (2000). Wireless capsule endoscopy. *Nature*, *405*(6785), 417.

Koulaouzidis, A., Iakovidis, D. K., Yung, D. E., Rondonotti, E., Kopylov, U., Plevris, J. N., et al. (2017). KID Project: An internet-based digital video atlas of capsule endoscopy for research purposes. *Endoscopy International Open*, *5*(06), E477–E483.

McAlindon, M. E., Ching, H.-L., Yung, D., Sidhu, R., & Koulaouzidis, A. (2016). Capsule endoscopy of the small bowel. *Annals of Translational Medicine*, *4*(19).

Moglia, A., Menciassi, A., Dario, P., & Cuschieri, A. (2009). Capsule endoscopy: Progress update and challenges ahead. *Nature Reviews Gastroenterology and Hepatology*, *6*(6), 353.

Spada, C., Hassan, C., Munoz-Navas, M., Neuhaus, H., Deviere, J., Fockens, P., et al. (2011). Second-generation colon capsule endoscopy compared with colonoscopy. *Gastrointestinal Endoscopy*, *74*(3), 581–589.

Part II
Technical Context

Chapter 3
Technical Context for Intelligent Systems in Colonoscopy

F. Javier Sánchez, Yael Tudela, Marina Riera, and Jorge Bernal

We define polyp presence detection as the capability of a given system to determine polyp presence in a given image. The expected output of a polyp detection system is a simple indication of if the system has predicted the presence of a polyp in the frame, without any kind of information of where it is in the image.

We extend this definition by denoting polyp localization as the capability of a system to indicate precisely where is the polyp within the image, in case it has determined such a presence. The majority of the methods published in the literature (which will be referenced in this chapter) use the terminology polyp detection to couple both polyp presence detection and polyp localization tasks.

Polyp segmentation can be described as the ability by which a given method is able to outline the polyp region in the image. While segmentation has no direct clinical task associated, it is commonly used as a prior stage in lesion classification methodologies.

We present in this chapter some of the current available methodologies that have been published for the before mentioned tasks as well as an indication of the current challenges that these methodologies have to deal with to provide a good performance.

3.1 State of the Art on Polyp Detection

Following the classification of computational approaches for polyp detection that was proposed in Bernal et al. (2017), we can divide existing methodologies in two big groups: handcrafted methods and machine learning ones.

F. J. Sánchez (✉) · Y. Tudela · M. Riera · J. Bernal
Computer Vision Center and Computer Science Department, Universitat Autònoma de Barcelona, 08193 Bellaterra (Cerdanyola del Vallès), Barcelona, Spain
e-mail: javier@cvc.uab.es

J. Bernal and A. Histace (eds.), *Computer-Aided Analysis of Gastrointestinal Videos*,
https://doi.org/10.1007/978-3-030-64340-9_3

Handcrafted methods are the ones that extract local features from the images and build a classifier (or detector) using those features as input. Local features are usually color descriptors (histograms) or pattern descriptors (key points) and are designed and tuned specifically to solve a concrete problem. This is one of the reasons why those methods normally don't generalize well across multiple datasets.

Machine learning algorithms are those which build a mathematical model based on patterns and inference from sample data, known as "training data". That way, they learn how to make predictions or decisions about a task, without being programmed for that specific task.

3.1.1 Handcrafted Methods

With respect to polyp detection and, to the best of our knowledge, the first method that tried to solve the colorectal polyp detection problem is the one from Karkanis et al. (2003), which was published on 2003. In their work, they tried to detect adenomatous tissues by color wavelet co-variance (CWC) of different regions from images and a step-wise linear discriminant analysis to classify the features.

Hwang et al. (2007) presented in 2007 a method that tried to exploit the common polyp shapes to detect the lesions on the images. They used watersheds to partially segment the images. Then they tried to fit ellipses into the watershed edge map and apply filters based on curve directions, curvature, and edge distance. Finally, they applied a threshold filter using the mean intensity value of the region. Also, they implemented inter-frame coherence based on ellipse distance between adjacent frames.

On 2012, Park et al. (2012) published a framework for polyp detection. First, they preprocessed the images removing the ones that weren't informative, and deinterlaced the others. Also they applied contrast equalization and removed specular regions using top-hat filters. From the informative images, they extracted features based on co-variance matrices from 5 to 10 sections of the frame and classified them into polyp/non-polyp. They used Conditional Random Fields (CRF) as a inter-frame coherence method, assuming that an adjacent frame should have a similar probability of being classified as the previous one.

Tajbakhsh et al. (2014) presented on 2014 a method that uses geometric constraints and intensity variations patterns (IVP) in the object boundaries in order to detect polyps in colonoscopy videos. Firstly they created an edge map from the image using Canny filters on RGB channels. Then, they refined this map by using IVP and computed a normalized DCT over multiple patches from the edges. Next, they classified those patches into five classes: polyp, lumen, vessel, reflections, and random. Also they computed the orientation of the patch for the ones classified as polyp. Finally they computed a voting map using these patches and orientations.

Bernal et al. (2015) proposed in 2015 a methodology based on a definition of model appearance for polyps. This model was built considering how colonoscopy images are acquired and it defined polyp boundaries by means of intensity valleys.

Once these are found, they created energy maps representing polyp presence in the image by integrating valley information in a way such complete, continuous, and circular structures are fostered. They were also the first to tackle the impact of other endoluminal structures in method performance: their results proved that the mitigation of specular highlights and blood vessels led to a overall increase in all considered metrics.

On 2015, Wang et al. (2015) presented Polyp-Alert a near real-time (10 frames per second) system for polyp detection in video. The system tried to identify if a previously detected edge map (obtained using Canny filter) is from a polyp or not. They extracted multiple features using edge cross-section profile (ECSP) related to the shape and length of the edges and also some features related to the texture and sizes of the enclosed regions. They consider polyp a region that are inside the range value for all the analyzed features. They also removed false positives regions using a tracking system. Their tracking system is based on optical-flow computation from a pyramid edge map and thresholding by a number of coincidences between contiguous frames.

On 2016, Geetha and Rajan (2016) published a method that combined three robust descriptors (LBP, DCT, and average color per channel) from different patches of an image. Then they fused the three different features to a common space and then used a decision tree, concretely J48, to make a detection for the frame.

3.1.2 Machine Learning Algorithms

Machine learning algorithms are those which build a mathematical model based on patterns and inference from sample data, known as "training data". That way, they learn how to make predictions or decisions about a task, without being programmed for that specific task

There have been many approaches that used classical machine learning paradigms (feature extractor + classifier, such as in the works of Angermann et al. 2017; Bae and Yoon 2015; Ameling et al. 2009 just to mention a few). The increasing availability of GPUs as well as the development of large public datasets has, as it has happened in many other research fields, led to the irruption of convolutional neural network methodologies to tackle polyp detection task.

There are various architectures mainly used regarding colorectal polyp detection. Those include one-stage methods such as SSD and YOLOv3, and two-stage methods: Faster R-CNN, Mask R-CNN, and the like.

On July 2018, Zheng et al. (2018) presented an application of a unified and real-time object detector based on You-Only-Look-Once (YOLO). Unlike the classification-based detectors, YOLO is a regression-based object detector which looks at the whole image once to perform the detection. It uses a single CNN simultaneously to predict bounding boxes as well as the class probabilities for the boxes. In addition, unlike sliding window and region proposal based detectors, YOLO looks at the entire image so it can encode contextual information during prediction which can reduce background mistakes.

On August 2018, Shin et al. (2018a, b) proposed a framework of conditional adversarial networks (conditional GAN) to increase the number of training samples by generating synthetic polyp images, as the lack of labeled polyp images for training is one of the major obstacles in this task. Generative Adversarial Networks (GAN) (Goodfellow et al. 2014) is a framework to generate artificial images by using the competitive way of two networks: generator and discriminator. Later, conditional GAN was proposed to control the labeling of the generated images. The authors propose training with synthetic images generated with conditional GAN, instead of applying simple image augmentation techniques, due to the large variation of polyps in terms of shape, scale, and color. Improved detection performance is achieved when the images are fed into a Faster R-CNN network.

On September 2018, Mo et al. (2018) made use of before mentioned Faster R-CNN framework for polyp detection. Faster-RCNN (Ren et al. 2015) is a detector that replaces handcrafted ROI selection step with a regional proposal network (RPN), and is much faster than the previous region proposal networks, thus achieving very competing results, and still being an efficient approach for clinical practice.

On October 2018, Qadir et al. (2020) proposed a method consisting of two phases: a region of interest (RoI) proposal by CNN-based object detector networks and a false positive (FP) reduction unit, which is important since CNNs have shown to be vulnerable to small perturbations and noise, thus sometimes missing the same polyp appearing in neighboring frames, producing a high number of false positives. In order to improve the overall performance of the CNN, the FP reduction unit exploits the bidirectional temporal coherence (among both previous and future frames) in video by integrating the RoIs in a set of consecutive frames, to make the final decision for each single frame. This showed how bidirectional temporal information is helpful in estimating polyp positions and accurately predict the FPs.

On January 2019, Kang and Gwak (2019) proposed an ensemble method for accurate polyp detection, consisting in the combination of two Mask R-CNN models with different backbone structures (ResNet50 and ResNet101) to enhance the performance and obtain a more accurate detection of the polyp. Mask R-CNN (He et al. 2017) is a two-stage network, and one of the best deep-learning models for segmentation, because it first detects targets in the image, and then produces the predicted mask for each detected target. In that sense, this model trades detection speed for a better segmentation of the polyp.

On April 2019, Zheng et al. (2019) proposed a method for polyp detection and tracking across following frames. The method, then, consisted of two parts. It initially detects and localizes polyps with a single frame object detector, such as U-Net. Then it used optical flow to track polyps and exploit temporal information. Also, to overcome tracking failure caused by camera motion, they trained a motion regression model, as well as a CNN, which is efficiently trained on-the-fly with the information of previous frames.

On May 2019, Liu et al. (2019) explored the application of single shot detector (SSD) framework, which can work at a very high frame rate, thus being suitable for clinic purposes. SSD is a one-stage method which uses a feed-forward CNN to produce a collection of fixed-size bounding boxes for each object from different feature maps. They also explored three different feature extractors: VGG16 (which is already integrated into SSD), ResNet50, and InceptionV3. The last two had to be specifically integrated into SSD by designing the multi-scale feature maps. Regarding the variety of polyp shape, size, and color, they found that InceptionV3 was the one to better capture those features, thus achieving the best performance among the three.

To close with this section, we present two tables summarizing the key points of the methodologies that have been described before (Tables 3.1 and 3.2).

Authors	Architecture	Novelty	Temporal coherence (yes/no)	Validation database	Metrics	Processing time
Zheng et al. (2018)	YOLO	Unified real-time object detector based on You-Only-Look-Once (YOLO) for polyp localization	None	CVC-ClinicDB, CVC-ColonDB (public), PWH-ColonDB (private)	Prec, Rec, F1, F2	Real-time
Shin et al. (2018b)	Faster-RCNN	Conditional GAN to increase the number of training samples by generating synthetic polyp images	None	CVC-Clinic, CVC-Clinic-VideoDB, ETIS-Larib (public), ASU-Mayo Clinic (no longer public)	Prec, Rec, Spec, Acc, F1, F2, MPT, RT, PDR	NA
Mo et al. (2018)	Faster-RCNN	VGG16 as the backbone followed by RPN and head networks	None	CVC-Clinic2015, CVC-Clinic2017, CVC-ColonDB, CVC-EndoSceneStill (public)	Prec, Rec, Acc, F1, F2, RT, MD (mean Euclidean distance)	17 fps
Qadir et al. (2020)	Faster-RCNN and SSD	RoI proposal followed by an FPs reduction unit integrating bidirectional temporal coherence in video	Integrates RoI in consecutive past and future frames, checking for FPs	CVC-Clinic, CVC-ClinicVideoDB (public), ASU-Mayo Clinic (no longer public)	Prec, Rec, Spec, F1	2.56 fps (Faster-RCNN), 30 fps (SSD)

Table 3.1 Summary of the main handcrafted methods

Authors	Novelty	Temporal coherence (yes/no)	Validation database	Metrics	Processing time
Karkanis et al. (2003)	Use of co-variance of second order in multiple bands wavelets as features and LDA as classifier	No	60 video sequences from private database	Specificity; recall	–
Hwang et al. (2007)	Use of watershed segmentation to find elliptical shapes and refinement exploiting common polyp shapes	Yes	27 video sequences form private database	Polyp detection rate	–
Park et al. (2012)	CRF as temporal coherence method that exploits the nature of colonoscopy videos	Yes	35 video sequences from private database	Specificity; recall	–
Tajbakhsh et al. (2014)	Novel patch descriptor that is robust to rotations and illumination changes followed by 2-stage classifier using a voting scheme	No	CVC-ColonDB	Precision; recall	–
Bernal et al. (2015)	Definition of a model of polyp appearance. Consideration of other endoluminal scene elements	No	CVC-ColonDB and CVC-ClinicDB	Precision; recall	10 s
Wang et al. (2015)	Edge features detector using features obtained from the ECSP. Tracking between frames using edge tracker	Yes	53 video sequences from private database	Recall; polyp detection rate	0.01 s per frame
Geetha and Rajan (2016)	Combined use of LBP, DCT and color as a robust local feature. Decision tree classifier using weighted features as inputs.	No	468 frames with polyp from a private database	Specificity; recall; F-score	–

Table 3.2 Summary of the main approaches using machine learning

Authors	Method	Novelty	Temporal coherence (yes/no)	Validation database	Metrics	Processing time
Liu et al. (2019)	SSD	Multi-scale feature maps integrated into SSD with different feature extractors: ResNet50, VGG16 and InceptionV3	None	CVC-ColonDB, CVC-ClinicDB, ETIS-Larib (public)	Prec, Rec, Spec, F1, F2	30–33 fps
Kang and Gwak (2019)	Mask-RCNN ensamble	Ensemble to combine two Mask R-CNN models (ResNet50 and ResNet101) for improved segmentation	None	CVC-ClinicDB, ETIS-Larib, CVC-ColonDB (public)	Prec, Rec, IU	NA
Zheng et al. (2019)	On-the-fly trained CNN	Fusion of a U-Net to detect polyps in single frame, and an algorithm for tracking the center of the polyp through following frames, using an optical-flow (OptCNN) trained on-the-fly with previous frames	Exploit temporal coherence for tracking a single polyp through following frames	CVC-VideoClinicDB (public)	Prec, Rec, F1, F2	NA

3.2 State of the Art on Polyp Segmentation

As for detection, polyp segmentation has also attracted the attention of several researchers during recent years. It is true that the number of related paper is significantly smaller than for the first task; this can be associated with the lack of large publicly available datasets or with the lack of direct clinical applicability of polyp segmentation. Nevertheless, we present in this section a brief recap of some of the most recent developments in the field.

Bernal et al. (2014) presented in 2014 their approach for polyp segmentation, which is a continuation of their work performed for polyp localization. In this case, they used the information provided by the intensity valleys image and the polyp localization energy map to create a first segmentation of the lesion. To remove outliers vertexes and to increase the smoothness of the final region, a median operator is applied. This is the first work tested on a public dataset. This work also tackles the impact of endoluminal scene objects in segmentation performance, showing again superior results when specular highlights and blood vessels are mitigated.

Vázquez et al. (2017) proposed in 2017 the first study on complete endoluminal scene segmentation (including polyps) using convolutional neural networks. In this case, the authors based their methodology on Fully Convolutional Networks (FCNs). They also studied the impact that data augmentation could have on the performance, as well as whether the performance of the main task (polyp segmentation) could be affected by the number of target classes to be segmented. Their results clearly outperformed state-of-the-art methods, showing that the use of deep-learning methods is a clear alternative to classical approaches.

One year later and also using as base architecture FCNs, Akbari et al. (2018) proposed a methodology which incorporates both a pre-processing and a post-processing stage. In the former, patch selection is performed to improve the candidates fed in the training stage. The result provided by the network is post-processed using Otsu thresholding and connected components analysis to improve the performance. The authors incorporated weights from Caffe to improve the training stage.

Last year, Qadir et al. (2019) presented their approach for polyp segmentation in which they trained a two-stage network (Mask R-CNN) using different CNN architectures (Resnet50, Resnet101 and InceptionResnetV2) for polyp segmentation. The authors show that the three different feature extractors that they propose do indeed compute different types of features due to differences in their number of layers and architectures. They propose an ensemble model to combine the outputs obtained in intermediate stages of the methods but in a way such models support each other when deemed necessary. Due to the lack of available images, they also tried to incorporate weights from pre-trained models such as VOC 2012 dataset, which led to an improvement in the overall performance.

Also in 2019, Kang and Gwak (2019) also proposed the use of Mask R-CNN for polyp segmentation. Similar to the previous work, an ensemble using different backbone structures (ResNet50 and ResNet101) was used to incorporate information gathered by different feature extractors, which also led to an improvement in the

Table 3.3 Summary of polyp segmentation methods

Authors	Method	Novelty	Validation database	Metrics	Processing time
Bernal et al. (2014)	Handcrafted	Mitigation of endoluminal scene elements	CVC-ColonDB	DICE, Jaccard	12 s
Vázquez et al. (2017)	FCNs	Use of several classes (polyp, lumen, specular)	CVC-ColonDB, CVC-ClinicDB	IoU, Acc	12 fps
Akbari et al. (2018)	FCNs	Use of pre and post-processing stage. Pre-trained on Caffe	CVC-ColonDB	Prec, Rec, Spec, DICE	N/A
Qadir et al. (2019)	Mask R-CNN	Ensemble of ResNet based architectures. Pre-trained on VOC 2012	CVC-ColonDB, CVC-ClinicDB, ETIS-Larib	Prec, Rec, DICE, Jaccard	N/A
Kang and Gwak (2019)	Mask R-CNN	Ensemble of ResNet based architectures. Pre-trained on COCO	CVC-ColonDB, CVC-ClinicDB, ETIS-Larib	Prec, Rec, IoU	N/A

overall performance. They also used pre-trained weights (in this case from COCO) due to the lack of large publicly available datasets.

Other base architectures have also been recently proposed, such as Generative Adversarial Networks (GANs) in the work of Poomeshwaran et al. (2019) or U-Net (Zhou et al. 2018) (Table 3.3).

3.3 Technical Challenges

3.3.1 Polyp Detection and Localization

A clinically useful automatic polyp detection methodology in colonoscopy has to deal with the in-vivo analysis of images acquired during a colonoscopy procedure. During the exploration, clinicians try to cover the majority of the colon wall to increase the likelihood of finding polyps; several protocols and guidelines are already defined to indicate clinicians how this exploration should be made. They include

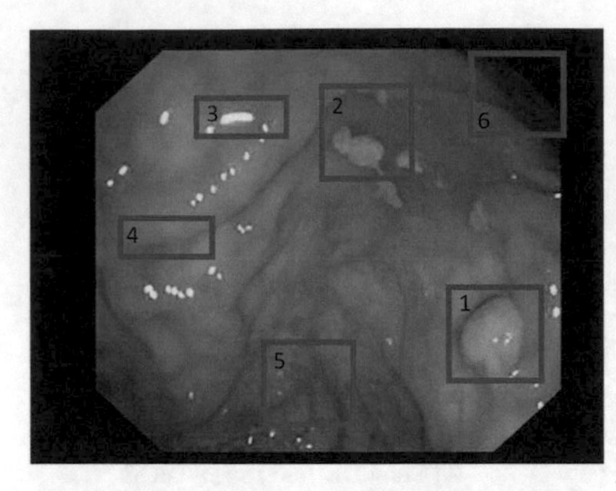

1. A polyp
2. Fecal particles
3. Specular highlights
4. Intestinal folds
5. Blood vessels
6. Luminal region

Fig. 3.1 Image showing a complete endoluminal scene with several elements on it

topics such as preparation quality to the need of reaching the cecum before starting the withdrawal stage. Even considering this useful guidelines and, as mentioned in the clinical introduction, still some polyps are missed. Therefore, the role of computational systems can be understood as not only finding those polyps that already appear in the images but also to guide clinicians to those areas that are suspicious to contain lesions.

Considering this, we could state that polyp detection presents several challenges. First, it is important to determine if the majority of the colon wall was observed during the exploration. Second, it is important to assess whether the quality of the images acquired is enough to be used by computational systems. Third and final, efficient polyp detection methods have to be developed. In this subsection we will focus on how to deal with this last challenge and we will link this with those problems that appear due to image quality issues.

A polyp can be characterized by means of its shape, color, and texture. Polyp visual appearance characterization has to be specific enough to differentiate them from other endoluminal scene elements, such as the ones shown in Fig. 3.1.

Paris classification (Van Doorn et al. 2015) determines the different shapes that a polyp can have. In the majority of the cases, polyps can be seen as protruding structures from the colon wall. Thus, a good characterization of these protruding elements can be a key for polyp detection, as it can provide false detections due to intestinal folds or fecal particles resulting for poor patient preparation. Moreover, this way of characterizing polyps is not valid for flat or depressed polyps. It also has to be considered that polyps visual appearance can vary due to the view of point.

With respect to polyps, they tend to appear reddish than abdominal wall. They could even have some blood particles in their surface. While this could be seen as a promising cue to aid in polyp detection, differentiation by color is a tough pathway as the difference relies in the hue more than in the color itself. Besides, this is not valid for all cases. For instance, polyps in their very early stages present colors very similar to the colon wall; these polyps are the most difficult to detect and, due to lengthy periods between interval colonoscopies, they could be one of the main causes of cancer development.

Finally, polyps do present a different texture from the colon wall. As Kudo pit pattern classification suggests (Kudo et al. 2001), these differences increase with the level of development of the lesion. While this classification paradigm is powerful for in-vivo histological prediction, it does have some specific technical constraints as it requires magnifying endoscopy and virtual chromoendoscopy, as well as High Definition endoscopy imaging. The use of these images requires more processing time and they are often downsampled to allow meeting real-time constraints, needed for a practical use in the exploration room.

As it can be seen, shape, color, and texture are three features that can help to characterize polyps but none of them alone is enough to cover all cases. All of them are affected by the quality of the images acquired during the exploration, which will be the focus of our next section.

3.3.1.1 Image Quality

The quality of the images acquired by the endoscopes is limited by the resolution, noise, movement, optical deformation, and other problems associated with the scene that has to be captured. These limitations affect the performance of automatic polyp detection and segmentation methods. We will see how each of the image quality limitations impact polyps visual features.

Endoscopy is non-invasive way to obtain images of the interior of the human body. Endoscopy tubes have at one or their tips all the instrumental needed to acquire images (camera, lighting source, and procedure instrumental), all designed with a high degree of miniaturization (Yabe 1990). With this configuration, endoscope illumination of the endoscope is frontal as the light comes from the same point where the camera is. Frontal illumination generates many specular reflections (Sánchez et al. 2017) over the aqueous surface of the colon. The size and position of these specular reflections could hinder those characteristics that allow the detection of polyps. Furthermore, these reflections are very unstable and their appearance change with small movements of the endoscope. This makes frame-by-frame polyp detection output very unstable; this can be mitigated by forcing the use of temporal integration techniques such as considering the response in consecutive frames to improve the results (Angermann et al. 2017). Reflections make it difficult to fully observe polyp shape, color, or texture, therefore equally affecting all visual characteristics of the polyps. Although there are methods to recover the contents below specular reflections, they are not that applicable in colonoscopy images as they also have to deal with inherent overexposure that could have removed key information from the colon wall.

Endoscopes use wide-angle optics in order to maximize the observed area of the colon and thus preventing any part of the colon wall from being inspected. It has to be noted that this also leads to a deformation of the image up to the point that the content of the corners of the image is removed as it could lead to misinterpretations of the scene. This geometric deformation invalidates the possibility of making accurate measurements and it is also the cause of the great variation in polyp appearance as it deviates from the center of the image, making it difficult for their characterization by means of shape features.

The use of wide-angle optics (Adler et al. 2012) reduces the resolution of the camera making each pixel occupy a larger area. Also, the area that a pixel occupies grows as we move away from the center of the image. This means that the details of the texture of a polyp can only be observed correctly in the center of the image, and even then, the captured detail of the texture will be insufficient due to the lack of resolution.

The miniaturization of the endoscope camera forces the use of small sensors that tend to present worse features than larger ones. Thus, the images captured by the endoscope are affected by noise introduced by image capture noise. Additionally, these sensors have low resolution, which has a special impact on the acquisition of texture details. On the one hand, smaller textures are difficult to distinguish from image noise. On the other hand, texture details could not be present at all due to the lack of resolution. Thus, texture details can only be properly observed in close-up views of polyp surface. Consequently, texture can hardly be used to detect those challenging polyps as, in those cases where enough texture quality information can be observed, the endoscopist would have already seen the polyp.

Endoscope manufacturers try to reduce the impact of using small sensors that generate poor quality images by applying aggressive image processing techniques. On the one hand, the sensors do not reach HD resolution (1920×1080 pixels), so they scale the image to display it on HD monitors. On the other hand, they aim to foster details captured in the images with the application of aggressive sharpening filters (Cao et al. 2011). While these filters do give a better visual appearance to the images, they do it at the expense of introducing halos which generate intensity ridges and valleys that were not in the raw sensor image. This means that, when detecting fine details in the images, it is difficult to be sure if they are real or they appear as a result of the processing that the manufacturer has applied to the images. In addition, the use of sharpening also emphasizes noise in images, which results in an even lower image resolution. All this artificial processing especially affects the texture and polyps contour detection.

Finally, in some cases, the endoscope sensor does not capture all the pixels in the image at the same time instant. For example, image acquisition might be based on interlaced television standards; in these cases, odd and even image lines are captured at different times. Other standards aim to improve image colorimetry by capturing three separate monochrome images with red, green, and blue lighting, which are then put together to obtain a single color image. This works well unless the endoscopy moves; in these cases, the images to be combined represent lightly different points of view. This produces artifacts in the image such as saw-tooth outlines (Faroudja and Swartz 1997) or colored reflections that make it difficult to extract the visual characteristics of the polyps.

3.3.1.2 Actual Ground Truth Limitations

Videos of endoscopic explorations are used to validate polyps detection methods. In these examinations, the endoscopist looks for polyps and when he/she finds them, he observes them carefully to decide what is the best action to take. Therefore, the videos that will be generated are not fully useful to test the capabilities of a polyp detection system as, once it is detected, the following frames will consist of close-ups views of the polyp that tend to be easy to detect.

To perform an appropriate validation of polyp detection methods, explorations should be recorded without further polyp analysis by means of the endoscopist. This is not realistic, as we are dealing with real patients that have to be diagnosed. One possible solution is to explore partially the colon and recording two different videos per part: one without clinician intervention and another one where he/she interacts with the lesion. This would result in an excessive procedure time and would lead to a saturation of the healthcare system. Taking this into account, performance metrics should not rely only on frame-based measurements. We will develop more on this in the specific Experimental Setup part of this book.

Current screening protocols could lead to certain biases in the appearance and typology of the polyps detected, since there are no representative examples of all the age strata of the population. This results in uneven ground truths that are not representative of the full range of polyps. Also, current available datasets are created by using lots of frames from very few different polyps, which could lead to the development of polyp detection methods that do not generalize well. Efforts have to be made to enlarge existing datasets with new and different examples.

3.3.2 Polyp Segmentation

The way polyp segmentation is seen, from a clinical application point of view, leads to its use in the analysis of still frames rather than on full sequences. This could alleviate real-time constraints and allow working with the maximum available image resolution. As we mentioned earlier, the direct application of polyp segmentation is to indicate the area of the colon wall occupied by the polyp. This information could be used to assist clinician in lesion removal tasks as well as to highlights those part of the image to be carefully inspected to obtain an in-vivo histology prediction.

As polyp segmentation can be done with still images, the system can select the highest quality image from all the sets of images that are being acquired. For instance, selection criteria could be based on choosing the image with the optimal focus and best exposure. This would allow to better observe the details of polyp boundary which, for sure, ease its segmentation. In this case, the segmentation method could also rely on the same features that we used for polyp detection (shape, color, and texture), inheriting the same issues related to image quality already mentioned. Fortunately, working with still images alleviates some of these problems, specially if the system is able to select the best quality image from a set of candidates.

The appearance of specular reflections in the image may cause that the segmentation method has to extrapolate the shape of the polyp if the reflection covers part of the polyp border. We should also consider that this problem occurs when the border is hardly noticeable, which happens when there is no change in color or texture at the polyp boundary. In this case, it is important to remember that a polyp can appear as a smooth protruding object in the colon wall, producing in this case just a smooth curvature on its border. This smooth change in curvature generates very weak gradients that can hardly be detected without applying a shape model. These gradients are hidden by the image's texture and noise, making it even more difficult to detect. In other cases, polyp boundary can be easily detected as it is highlighted by a large curvature or fold on the surface that can easily be detected as a valley in the image.

With respect to dataset availability, the number of publicly available datasets is very small. Existing ones do not cover a great number of different polyps and, the largest ones (in terms of number of images) have low resolution. Efforts have to be made to enlarge these datasets both in number of different polyps (the use of video datasets in this case does not appear specially useful) and quality of the image. The use of HD-based datasets could be used for both polyp segmentation and classification tasks.

References

Adler, A., Aminalai, A., Aschenbeck, J., Drossel, R., Mayr, M., Scheel, M., et al. (2012). Latest generation, wide-angle, high-definition colonoscopes increase adenoma detection rate. *Clinical Gastroenterology and Hepatology*, *10*(2), 155–159.

Akbari, M., Mohrekesh, M., Nasr-Esfahani, E., Soroushmehr, S. R., Karimi, N., Samavi, S., et al. (2018). Polyp segmentation in colonoscopy images using fully convolutional network. In *2018 40th Annual International Conference of the IEEE Engineering in Medicine and Biology Society (EMBC)* (pp. 69–72). IEEE.

Ameling, S., Wirth, S., Paulus, D., Lacey, G., & Vilarino, F. (2009). Texture-based polyp detection in colonoscopy. *Bildverarbeitung für die Medizin 2009* (pp. 346–350). Berlin: Springer.

Angermann, Q., Bernal, J., Sánchez-Montes, C., Hammami, M., Fernández-Esparrach, G., Dray, X., et al. (2017). Towards real-time polyp detection in colonoscopy videos: Adapting still frame-based methodologies for video sequences analysis. *Computer assisted and robotic endoscopy and clinical image-based procedures* (pp. 29–41). Berlin: Springer.

Bae, S.-H., & Yoon, K.-J. (2015). Polyp detection via imbalanced learning and discriminative feature learning. *IEEE Transactions on Medical Imaging*, *34*(11), 2379–2393.

Bernal, J., Núñez, J. M., Sánchez, F. J., & Vilariño, F. (2014). Polyp segmentation method in colonoscopy videos by means of MSA-DOVA energy maps calculation. In *Workshop on Clinical Image-Based Procedures* (pp. 41–49). Springer.

Bernal, J., Sánchez, F. J., Fernández-Esparrach, G., Gil, D., Rodríguez, C., & Vilariño, F. (2015). WM-DOVA maps for accurate polyp highlighting in colonoscopy: Validation vs. saliency maps from physicians. *Computerized Medical Imaging and Graphics*, *43*, 99–111.

Bernal, J., Tajkbaksh, N., Sánchez, F. J., Matuszewski, B. J., Chen, H., Yu, L., et al. (2017). Comparative validation of polyp detection methods in video colonoscopy: Results from the MICCAI 2015 endoscopic vision challenge. *IEEE Transactions on Medical Imaging*, *36*(6), 1231–1249.

Cao, G., Zhao, Y., Ni, R., & Kot, A. C. (2011). Unsharp masking sharpening detection via overshoot artifacts analysis. *IEEE Signal Processing Letters*, *18*(10), 603–606.

Faroudja, Y. C., & Swartz, P. D. (1997). Suppression of sawtooth artifacts in an interlace-to-progressive converted signal. US Patent 5,625,421.

Geetha, K., & Rajan, C. (2016). Automatic colorectal polyp detection in colonoscopy video frames. *Asian Pacific Journal of Cancer Prevention*, *17*(11), 4869.

Goodfellow, I. J., Pouget-Abadie, J., Mirza, M., Xu, B., Warde-Farley, D., Ozair, S., et al. (2014). Generative adversarial networks.

He, K., Gkioxari, G., Dollör, P., & Girshick, R. (2017). Mask R-CNN.

Hwang, S., Oh, J., Tavanapong, W., Wong, J., & Groen, P. (2007). Polyp detection in colonoscopy video using elliptical shape feature. In *Proceedings - International Conference on Image Processing, ICIP* (Vol. 2, pp. II–465).

Kang, J., & Gwak, J. (2019). Ensemble of instance segmentation models for polyp segmentation in colonoscopy images. *IEEE Access*, *7*, 26440–26447.

Karkanis, S. A., Iakovidis, D. K., Maroulis, D. E., Karras, D. A., & Tzivras, M. (2003). Computer-aided tumor detection in endoscopic video using color wavelet features. *IEEE Transactions on Information Technology in Biomedicine*, *7*, 141–152.

Kudo, S., Rubino, C., Teixeira, C., Kashida, H., & Kogure, E. (2001). Pit pattern in colorectal neoplasia: Endoscopic magnifying view. *Endoscopy*, *33*(04), 367–373.

Liu, M., Jiang, J., & Wang, Z. (2019). Colonic polyp detection in endoscopic videos with single shot detection based deep convolutional neural network. *IEEE Access*, *7*, 75058–75066.

Mo, X., Tao, K., Wang, Q., & Wang, G. (2018). An efficient approach for polyps detection in endoscopic videos based on faster R-CNN. In *2018 24th International Conference on Pattern Recognition (ICPR)*.

Park, S. Y., Sargent, D., Spofford, I., Vosburgh, K. G., & A-Rahim, Y. (2012). A colon video analysis framework for polyp detection. *IEEE Transactions on Biomedical Engineering*, *59*, 1408–1418.

Poomeshwaran, J., Santhosh, K. S., Ram, K., Joseph, J., & Sivaprakasam, M. (2019). Polyp segmentation using generative adversarial network. In *2019 41st Annual International Conference of the IEEE Engineering in Medicine and Biology Society (EMBC)* (pp. 7201–7204). IEEE.

Qadir, H. A., Shin, Y., Solhusvik, J., Bergsland, J., Aabakken, L., & Balasingham, I. (2019). Polyp detection and segmentation using mask R-CNN: Does a deeper feature extractor CNN always perform better? In *2019 13th International Symposium on Medical Information and Communication Technology (ISMICT)* (pp. 1–6). IEEE.

Qadir, H. A., Balasingham, I., Solhusvik, J., Bergsland, J., Aabakken, L., & Shin, Y. (2020). Improving automatic polyp detection using CNN by exploiting temporal dependency in colonoscopy video. *IEEE Journal of Biomedical and Health Informatics*, *24*(1), 180–193.

Ren, S., He, K., Girshick, R., & Sun, J. (2015). Faster R-CNN: Towards real-time object detection with region proposal networks. In *Advances in Neural Information Processing Systems* (pp. 91–99).

Sánchez, F. J., Bernal, J., Sánchez-Montes, C., de Miguel, C. R., & Fernández-Esparrach, G. (2017). Bright spot regions segmentation and classification for specular highlights detection in colonoscopy videos. *Machine Vision and Applications*, *28*(8), 917–936.

Shin, Y., Qadir, H. A., Aabakken, L., Bergsland, J., & Balasingham, I. (2018a). Automatic colon polyp detection using region based deep CNN and post learning approaches. *IEEE Access*, *6*, 40950–40962.

Shin, Y., Qadir, H. A., & Balasingham, I. (2018b). Abnormal colon polyp image synthesis using conditional adversarial networks for improved detection performance. *IEEE Access*, *6*, 56007–56017.

Tajbakhsh, N., Gurudu, S. R., & Liang, J. (2014). Automatic polyp detection using global geometric constraints and local intensity variation patterns. In *Medical Image Computing and Computer-Assisted Intervention*.

Van Doorn, S. C., Hazewinkel, Y., East, J. E., Van Leerdam, M. E., Rastogi, A., Pellisé, M., et al. (2015). Polyp morphology: An interobserver evaluation for the Paris classification among international experts. *American Journal of Gastroenterology*, *110*(1), 180–187.

Vázquez, D., Bernal, J., Sánchez, F. J., Fernández-Esparrach, G., López, A. M., Romero, A., et al. (2017). A benchmark for endoluminal scene segmentation of colonoscopy images. *Journal of Healthcare Engineering, 2017*.

Wang, Y., Tavanapong, W., Wong, J., Oh, J. H., & de Groen, P. C. (2015). Polyp-Alert: Near real-time feedback during colonoscopy. *Computer Methods and Programs in Biomedicine, 120*, 164–179.

Yabe, H. (1990). Endoscope with a detachable observation unit at its distal end. US Patent 4,895,138.

Zheng, Y., Zhang, R., Yu, R., Jiang, Y., Mak, T. W. C., Wong, S. H., et al. (2018). Localisation of colorectal polyps by convolutional neural network features learnt from white light and narrow band endoscopic images of multiple databases. In *2018 40th Annual International Conference of the IEEE Engineering in Medicine and Biology Society (EMBC)*.

Zheng, H., Chen, H., Huang, J., Li, X., Han, X., & Yao, J. (2019). Polyp tracking in video colonoscopy using optical flow with an on-the-fly trained CNN. In *2019 IEEE 16th International Symposium on Biomedical Imaging (ISBI 2019)*.

Zhou, Z., Siddiquee, M. M. R., Tajbakhsh, N., & Liang, J. (2018). UNet++: A nested U-Net architecture for medical image segmentation. *Deep learning in medical image analysis and multimodal learning for clinical decision support* (pp. 3–11). Berlin: Springer.

Chapter 4
Technical Context for Wireless Capsule Endoscopy Image Analysis

Aymeric Histace

4.1 WCE and Small Bowel

As said before, WCE has rapidly become the standard minimally invasive method for visualization of the Small Bowel (SB) which is highly difficult to reach using classic endoscopy techniques like enteroscopy.

SB is part of the intestines. The intestines are a long, continuous tube running from the stomach to the anus. Most absorption of nutrients and water happen in the intestines. The intestines include the SB, colon, and rectum (Fig. 4.1).

SB is about 20 feet long and about an inch in diameter. Its job is to absorb most of the nutrients from what we eat and drink. Velvety tissue lines the small intestine, which is divided into the duodenum, jejunum, and ileum.

Problems with the small intestine can include

- Bleeding
- Celiac disease
- Crohn's disease
- Infections
- Intestinal cancer
- Intestinal obstruction
- Irritable bowel syndrome
- Ulcers, such as peptic ulcer.

A. Histace (✉)
ENSEA, ETIS UMR 8051 (CY Paris Cergy University, ENSEA, CNRS),
6 av. du Ponceau, 95014 Cergy, France
e-mail: aymeric.histace@ensea.fr

J. Bernal and A. Histace (eds.), *Computer-Aided Analysis of Gastrointestinal Videos*,
https://doi.org/10.1007/978-3-030-64340-9_4

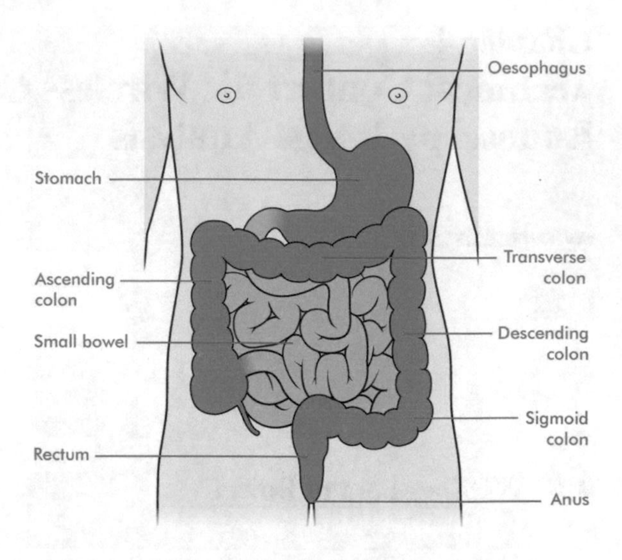

Fig. 4.1 Intestines morphology

4.2 Vascular and Inflammatory Lesions in SB

In the context of GIANA challenge, a focus on two classic intestinal types of lesions was proposed because of their prevalence in WCE exam indication:

- Gastrointestinal angiodysplasia (GIA)
- inflammatory Bowel lesions (IBL).

GIA is an acquired vascular malformation defined as a clearly demarcated, bright-red, flat lesion, consisting of tortuous and clustered capillary dilatation, within the mucosal layer (Leenhardt et al. 2018). GIAs are the most common small bowel (SB) vascular lesions and are associated with a risk of gastrointestinal bleeding (Becq et al. 2017).

IBL is a generic term used to describe disorders that involve chronic inflammation of the digestive tract (Bharadwaj et al. 2018). Types of IBL include ulcerative colitis that cause long-lasting inflammation and sores (ulcers) and Crohn's disease characterized by inflammation of the lining of the digestive tract, which often spreads deep into affected tissues.

4.3 Remaining Challenges

Despite the fact that WCE has shown a real impact for lesion detections in SB, limitations still remain (Goel et al. 2014) (Figs. 4.2 and 4.3):

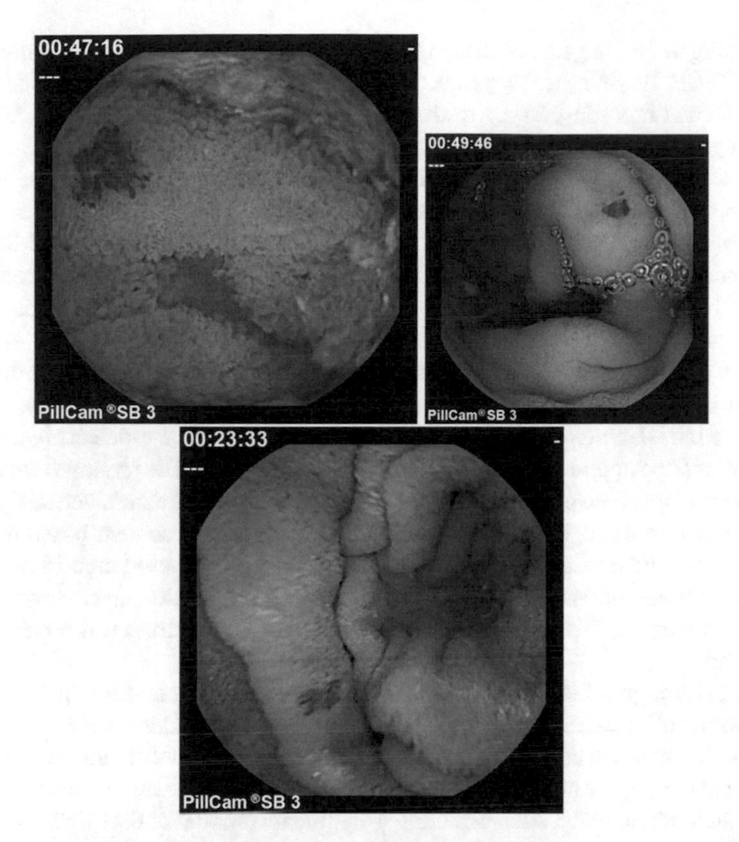

Fig. 4.2 Some examples of WCE images presenting with GIA

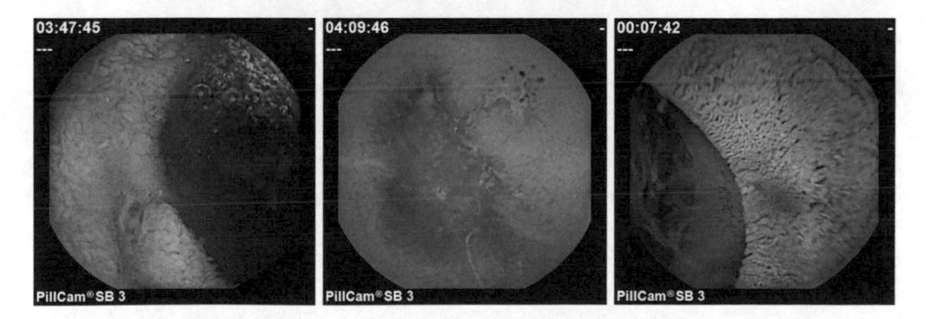

Fig. 4.3 Some examples of WCE images presenting with IBL

- missed lesions due to reader error or technical malfunction;
- unable to obtain biopsies or perform therapeutic interventions;
- the position of the capsule cannot be accurately controlled;
- potentially obstructed views from inadequate bowel preparation;
- subjectivity of interpretation of images by the observer.

To mitigate the impacts of these limitations, AI applications are emerging in the field of WCE. In the next few years, automated software should be able to facilitate more efficient reporting. Many studies have been conducted in order to establish a cleansing score for SB-CE quality preparation. Different approaches have focused on the abundance of bubbles (Pietri et al. 2018), the red over green color (Van Weyenberg et al. 2011; Ali et al. 2018), as well as the quality of bowel preparation in colon capsule endoscopy (Becq et al. 2018). Algorithms based on machine learning approaches have also been developed to detect SB lesions (Fan et al. 2018; Leenhardt et al. 2019) and recently it has been proposed to scale-up the process to be able to bring it to the level of Software as a Service (SaaS).

More precisely, an AI-based framework for Supporting large-scale automated analysis of WCE was proposed in Giordano et al. (2019). More precisely, authors introduced an AI-based computational framework which is able to detect eight classes of lesion and to support large-scale analysis of VCE videos. The proposed system, in particular, supports all processing stages, from video upload to automated analysis for lesion detection through a deep learning-based method, to a content-based retrieval system to facilitate diagnosis, to report generation. The proposed algorithm reports a mean accuracy of 94.4% considering a 8-lesion classification task. Nevertheless, the dataset used for this study is not available and the ground truth was not explicitly illustrated.

Thus, although AI in endoscopy remains very promising, it still requires further research and clinical trials to be validated in daily clinical practice, and a strong need for large annotated databases, at the segmentation level, not only at the classification one, is still of primary interest. To this aim, GIANA challenge was the first to propose a collection of annotated data providing a significant amount of data with a focus on both types of lesions that were described above.

4.4 Conclusions

In conclusion, the GIANA database aims to promote development of CAD reading in SB-WCE. It represents an opportunity to design fully automated software for detection of all SB lesions to facilitate and improve the future of WCE reading, reviewing, and reporting.

References

Ali, E. A., Histace, A., Camus, M., Gerometta, R., Becq, A., Pietri, O., et al. (2018). Development and validation of a computed assessment of cleansing score for evaluation of quality of small-bowel visualization in capsule endoscopy. *Endoscopy International Open*, *6*(06), E646–E651.

Becq, A., Rahmi, G., Perrod, G., & Cellier, C. (2017). Hemorrhagic angiodysplasia of the digestive tract: Pathogenesis, diagnosis, and management. *Gastrointestinal Endoscopy*, *86*(5), 792–806.

Becq, A., Histace, A., Camus, M., Nion-Larmurier, I., Ali, E. A., Pietri, O., et al. (2018). Development of a computed cleansing score to assess quality of bowel preparation in colon capsule endoscopy. *Endoscopy International Open*, *6*(07), E844–E850.

Bharadwaj, S., Narula, N., Tandon, P., & Yaghoobi, M. (2018). Role of endoscopy in inflammatory bowel disease. *Gastroenterology Report*, *6*(2), 75–82.

Fan, S., Xu, L., Fan, Y., Wei, K., & Li, L. (2018). Computer-aided detection of small intestinal ulcer and erosion in wireless capsule endoscopy images. *Physics in Medicine and Biology*, *63*(16), 165001.

Giordano, D., Murabito, F., Palazzo, S., Pino, C., & Spampinato, C. (2019). An AI-based framework for supporting large scale automated analysis of video capsule endoscopy. In *2019 IEEE EMBS International Conference on Biomedical and Health Informatics (BHI)* (pp. 1–4). IEEE.

Goel, R. M., Patel, K. V., Borrow, D., & Anderson, S. (2014). Video capsule endoscopy for the investigation of the small bowel: Primary care diagnostic technology update. *British Journal of General Practice*, *64*(620), 154–156.

Leenhardt, R., Li, C., Koulaouzidis, A., Cavallaro, F., Cholet, F., Eliakim, A. R., et al. (2018). Sa1028 terminology and description of vascular lesions in small bowel capsule endoscopy: An international Delphi consensus statement. *Gastrointestinal Endoscopy*, *87*(6), AB149–AB150.

Leenhardt, R., Vasseur, P., Li, C., Saurin, J. C., Rahmi, G., Cholet, F., et al. (2019). A neural network algorithm for detection of GI angiectasia during small-bowel capsule endoscopy. *Gastrointestinal Endoscopy*, *89*(1), 189–194.

Pietri, O., Rezgui, G., Histace, A., Camus, M., Nion-Larmurier, I., Li, C., et al. (2018). Development and validation of an automated algorithm to evaluate the abundance of bubbles in small bowel capsule endoscopy. *Endoscopy International Open*, *6*(04), E462–E469.

Van Weyenberg, S. J., De Leest, H. T., & Mulder, C. J. (2011). Description of a novel grading system to assess the quality of bowel preparation in video capsule endoscopy. *Endoscopy*, *43*(05), 406–411.

Part III
Methodologies

Chapter 5
Combination of Color-Based Segmentation, Markov Random Fields and Multilayer Perceptron

Pedro Miguel Vieira, Nuno Renato Freitas, Carla Rolanda, and Carlos Santo Lima

5.1 Motivation

Angioectasias are lesions characterized by specific features, related to the color and shape. These lesions have a cherry red appearance, due to the nature of its origin (inflammation of blood vessels); and usually are characterized with a circular shape. As was previously reported, CIELab color has high efficiency in differentiating colors in an image (Connolly and Fleiss 1997). This color space is composed of three different channels: L represents the lightness information that goes from 0 (black) to 100 (diffuse white), and the components a and b represent the color-opponent dimensions. Negative values of channel a indicate green and positive indicate magenta (adequate for the detection of red color); and negative values of b indicate blue and positive indicate yellow (Weatherall and Coombs 1992). Since the red color in these lesions is easily spotted in the middle of the gastrointestinal tissue, CIELab was the chosen color space for processing the lesions. A pre-processing was included to overcome some problems with high values of the component a that do not represent a red area on the tissue. This step was designed by observation of a high number of images, leading to the understanding that certain areas of the images (usually near bubbles) could lead the segmentation step to fail. As was already shown in a previous work of the authors (Vieira et al. 2016), these types of lesions can be separated from the normal tissue by using probabilistic segmentation methods, as the Maximum A Posteriori (MAP) approach. This method was complemented with the use of Markov Random Fields (MRF) to improve the border definition. Because the segmentation

P. M. Vieira (✉) · N. R. Freitas · C. S. Lima
CMEMS-UMinho Research Unit, Campus de Azurém - Universidade do Minho, Guimarães, Portugal
e-mail: pmpvieira@gmail.com

C. Rolanda
ICVS/3Bs - PT Government Associate Laboratory, Braga/Guimarães, Portugal

Department of Gastroenterology, Hospital de Braga, Braga, Portugal

J. Bernal and A. Histace (eds.), *Computer-Aided Analysis of Gastrointestinal Videos*,
https://doi.org/10.1007/978-3-030-64340-9_5

used was based on probability approaches, the authors decided to use statistical features to characterize the tissue and consequently to classify the images as having angioectasia lesions or not.

5.2 Methodology

This method can be divided into three different subsections: Image Pre-Processing, Segmentation and finally Features Extraction + Classification.

5.2.1 Pre-processing

The pre-processing is made so the angioectasia lesions can be highlighted in the image when compared to the rest of the tissue. Due to the reddish appearance of angioectasias, the choice of color space was CIELab; in this specific space, high values of the component a represent the red color (Weatherall and Coombs 1992). Nevertheless, due to specific noise of WCE exams (e.g., bubbles), not only these lesions appear highlighted in the images. So, the following algorithm was applied to the images. Let C be an RGB image with a $M \times N$ size and D the corresponding image in CIELab color space. $C^k(i, j)$ and $D^l(i, j)$ represent the correspondent pixel in the component $k = R, G, B$ and $l = L, a, b$, respectively, and with the coordinates $i = 1, 2, \ldots, M$ and $j = 1, 2, \ldots, N$. In this algorithm (Algorithm 5.1), the pixels that present values of green or blue components lower than a chosen threshold (δ) are replaced by an average of a neighboring region (with a variable size) centered in that pixel ($\aleph\{D^l(i, j)\}$).

Algorithm 5.1 Pre-processing algorithm

1: **for** each pixel (i, j) **do**
2:     **if** $C^G(i, j) < \delta$ or $C^B(i, j) < \delta$ **then**
3:         $D^a(i, j) \leftarrow \aleph\{D^a(i, j)\}$
4:         Break
5:     **end if**
6: **end for**

After this step, channel a of the images will have the regions with angioectasia highlighted. After this, the segmentation step will be applied.

5.2.2 Segmentation

The segmentation is based on a Maximum A Posteriori (MAP) approach by using the Expectation-Maximization (EM) algorithm (Vieira et al. 2016, 2019). A modified MRF, with a weighted boundary function, was included for spatial context modeling purposes.

The segmentation module uses a statistical classification based on Bayes rule. This rule indicates how the posterior probability of each class is calculated. MAP is computed for all classes and each pixel is assigned to the class with maximum MAP. Class conditional probability density function is usually assigned to the Gaussian function, being the observations modeled as a Gaussian mixture whose parameters can be iteratively estimated by using the EM algorithm.

The most appropriate parameters of the GMM are then estimated according to the Maximum Likelihood (ML) criterion (Zhang et al. 2001). Regarding the a priori probability, this has a precise meaning in the model regarding data partition over all classes; however, it is frequently used as a spatial regularizer by capturing neighboring information, not taken into consideration in the Gaussian mixture model that models pixel intensities as random variables which are independent and identically distributed. Neighborhood information can be modeled by Markov Random Fields (MRFs). MRF models have the ability of capturing neighborhood information to improve a priori probabilities $p(\omega)$. An image can be considered as a random field, or a collection of random variables $(\Omega = \Omega_1, \ldots, \Omega_N)$ that are defined on the set S. Using Gibbs Random Field (GRF), the a priori class probability can be assigned such as

$$P(\omega) = \frac{1}{Z} \exp\left(\frac{-U(\omega)}{T}\right) \tag{5.1}$$

$$Z = \sum_{\omega} exp\left(-\frac{U(\omega)}{T}\right) \tag{5.2}$$

In this equation, the constant T represents the temperature and controls the level of peaking in the probability density, and the quantity Z is a normalizing constant which guarantees that $p(\omega)$ is always between zero and one. $U(\omega)$ is an energy function and is obtained by summing all functions $V(\omega)$ (clique potential) over all C possible cliques. A clique is defined as a grouping of pixels in a neighborhood system, such that the grouping includes pixels that are neighbors of another in the same system.

The Hammersley–Clifford theorem defines that if and only if a random field Ω on S is a MRF with respect to neighborhood system $\mathcal{N}$, then Ω is a GRF on S with respect to a neighborhood system $\mathcal{N}$. This fact allows to convert the conditional probability as a Markovianity condition of a MRF to the non-conditional probability of a Gibbs distribution of Eq. (5.1).

To compute the estimation of $p(\omega)$, the energy function used was based on Van Leemput et al. (1999):

$$U(\omega_j) = \sum_k \beta_k . l_{k,j} \quad (5.3)$$

In Eq. (5.3), k is the direction (in this case it can be horizontal or vertical) and $l_{k,j}$ is the Dirac impulse function in such a way that $U(\omega_j)$ depends on the count of pixels in neighborhood that do not belong to class j.

Usually, in practice, models are considered as isotropic, so the amount of variables to estimate is strongly decreased, becoming in this case β_k a constant. However, pixels near the borders are sometimes wrongly classified in the Gaussian Mixture especially due to the partial volume effect. Therefore, using the β_k parameter to model intensity differences in neighborhood pixels in order to reinforce border conditions has been used in several works where several functions have been suggested. The main idea is to set β_k in such a way that a direct interference on border location is achieved. Heuristically we want to avoid class j under situations of high variance that usually appear near borders, even if a large number of pixels belong to class j. Under relative smooth conditions the border can also be present and can be detected by pixel intensity variations which occur at corners of small structures. Some tests were conducted in order to compute β_k for pixels on and near the border of several angioectasias and the approximated function given by Eq. (5.4) was used as follows:

$$\beta_k = \frac{\sigma_k}{1 + \exp\left(-\sigma_k \frac{\sum_i^n |I_i - I_c| . \mathrm{dist}(I_i, I_c)}{n}\right)} \quad (5.4)$$

In Eq. (5.4), β_k is dependent on the difference of intensities ($|I_i - I_c|$) of the neighbor in the direction k, but also of the distance between the pixel in the center and the neighboring pixel (dist(I_i, I_c)). The term σ is the standard deviation of the neighboring used in this case and presented in Fig. 5.1.

This energy function uses a 2D-neighboring system of 8 pixels that can be seen in Fig. 5.1, where the darker pixel is the current observation.

With all the previous steps followed, the process now is to find the best parameters. This is done in an iterative manner, proceeding as follows:

1. Initialization of parameters, which in this case was done by using K-means algorithm

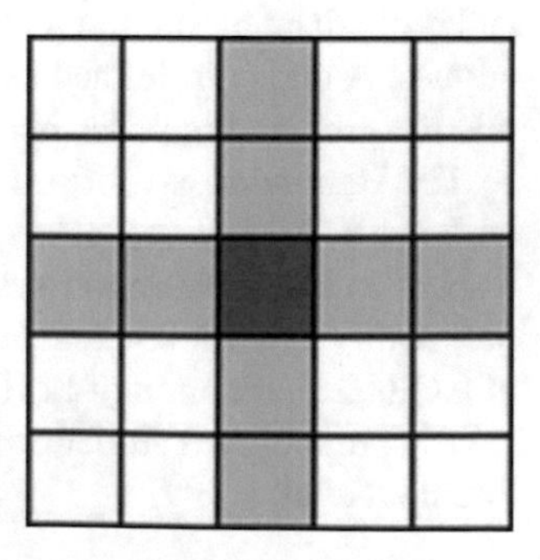

Fig. 5.1 Neighborhood system of 8 pixels used

2. E-step (expectation): calculation of likelihood of each sample for each class
3. M-step (maximization): find maximum likelihood value and recalculate the parameters

Steps 2 and 3 are repeated until convergence is achieved.

After the EM algorithm, a post-processing step was also included. This was done to improve the segmentation result since

1. isolated pixels are sometimes selected as abnormal region,
2. sharp and irregular edges appear in some lesions,
3. some pixels are included in the lesion class, but are in fact belonging to the normal class.

These problems are overcome with the following solutions:

1. Opening operation: using a small structuring element, the regions that consist of isolated pixels will disappear from the binary image.
2. Closing operation: using the same structuring element, smoothing the edges for both directions.
3. Shape analysis: because angioectasias are circular regions, connected components algorithm was applied, and lesions with a ratio between major and minor axis length superior than 3 were removed.

5.3 Feature Extraction + Classification

The output of the segmentation module described previously can have three different results:

1. after post-processing step, only one region exists in the image.
2. the image is divided into two different regions (one of them contains an angioectasia lesion),
3. the image is divided in two different regions (none of them contains an angioectasia lesion),

With situation 1, the image is classified as normal since no significant differences are found in channel a (so, different classes are not considered under the constraint of contiguous minimum area). When situation 2 or 3 happens, the classification module is necessary so the regions can be classified as normal or abnormal. This classification module needs features to feed it, that are extracted from both regions. This approach models the difference between both regions, in order to improve robustness against environmental conditions (related to device and subject changes). In fact, light characteristics may vary among different devices while tissue color may vary among different subjects.

Since the segmentation of the images was done based on the statistical distribution of the intensities, the features chosen were different statistical features that together

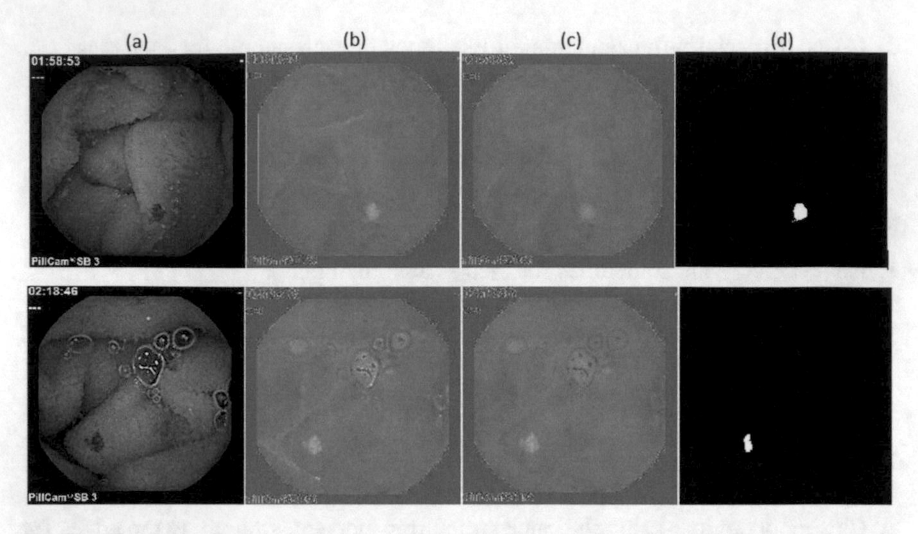

Fig. 5.2 Two examples of results with training images. **a** Original image. **b** Component a from CIELab. **c** Component a from CIELab after pre-processing step. **d** Segmentation result

can represent these distributions. In the current work, two different measures were computed (mean and variance), using the following expressions:

$$\mu = E\{X\} = \frac{1}{N}\sum_{i}^{N} x_i \tag{5.5}$$

$$\sigma^2 = E\{(X-\mu)^2\} = \frac{1}{N}\sum_{i}^{N}(x_i-\mu)^2 \tag{5.6}$$

All the features (from the different channels and different regions) were used as input to a Multilayer Perceptron (MLP) classifier with 1 hidden layer of 5 neurons. The output of the classifier is the presence or not of angioectasia tissue in each frame.

5.4 Results

Figure 5.2 shows some examples of results of the application of the proposed methodology over WCE images from GIANA 2017 dataset.

References

Connolly, C., & Fleiss, T. (1997). A study of efficiency and accuracy in the transformation from RGB to CIELAB color space. *IEEE Transactions on Image Processing*, *6*(7), 1046–1048.

Van Leemput, K., Maes, F., Vandermeulen, D., & Suetens, P. (1999). Automated model-based tissue classification of MR images of the brain. *IEEE Transactions on Medical Imaging*, *18*, 897–908.

Vieira, P. M., Gonçalves, B., Gonçalves, C. R., & Lima, C. S. (2016). Segmentation of angiodysplasia lesions in WCE images using a map approach with Markov random fields. In *2016 38th Annual International Conference of the IEEE Engineering in Medicine and Biology Society (EMBC)* (pp. 1184–1187). IEEE.

Vieira, P. M., Silva, C. P., Costa, D., Vaz, I. F., Rolanda, C., & Lima, C. S. (2019). Automatic segmentation and detection of small bowel angioectasias in WCE images. *Annals of Biomedical Engineering*, *47*, 1446–1462.

Weatherall, I. L., & Coombs, B. D. (1992). Skin color measurements in terms of CIELAB color space values. *Journal of Investigative Dermatology*, *99*(4), 468–473.

Zhang, Y., Brady, M., & Smith, S. (2001). Segmentation of brain MR images through a hidden Markov random field model and the expectation-maximization algorithm. *IEEE Transactions on Medical Imaging*, *20*(1), 45–57.

Chapter 6
Hand Crafted Method: ROI Selection and Texture Description

Orlando Chuquimia, Bertrand Granado, Xavier Dray, and Andrea Pinna

6.1 Motivation

The method presented here had been developed to be integrated in a SoC[1] implemented in a WCE [2] (Swain 2003). Its goal is to give a WCE the capacity to detect the polyps inside the colon (Orlando et al. 2017). To do that we need to take into account all non-functional constraints of an embedded system: real-time execution, energy budget, and limited area.

This method is inspired from the psychovisual two phases methodology used by a physician when doing a colonoscopic examination:

1. the first phase is the selection of the regions of interest (ROI), this phase is done using shape features.
2. the second phase is the polyp detection in an ROI and the follow-up of this ROI.

Based on this methodology, we propose a four-stage method visible in Fig: 6.1. The stages of our method are

1. **ROI selection stage**: in this stage, suspect regions that contain circular/elliptical shapes are selected and become ROI. These shapes could be a polyp. To do so, we apply the Hough Transform algorithm (Karargyris and Bourbakis 2011, 2009; Romain et al. 2013; Mamonov et al. 2014) on two color models.
2. **ROI follow-up stage**: in this stage, each ROI, validated as $class1$, is followed. The follow-up processing is based on a motion estimation method to determine where the ROI should be.

[1] System on Chip.
[2] Wireless Capsule Endoscopy.

O. Chuquimia (✉) · B. Granado · A. Pinna
LIP6, Sorbonne University, 4 place Jussieu, 75252 Paris, France
e-mail: orlando.chuquimia@lip6.fr

X. Dray
Saint-Antoine Hospital, APHP & Sorbonne University, Paris, France

J. Bernal and A. Histace (eds.), *Computer-Aided Analysis of Gastrointestinal Videos*,
https://doi.org/10.1007/978-3-030-64340-9_6

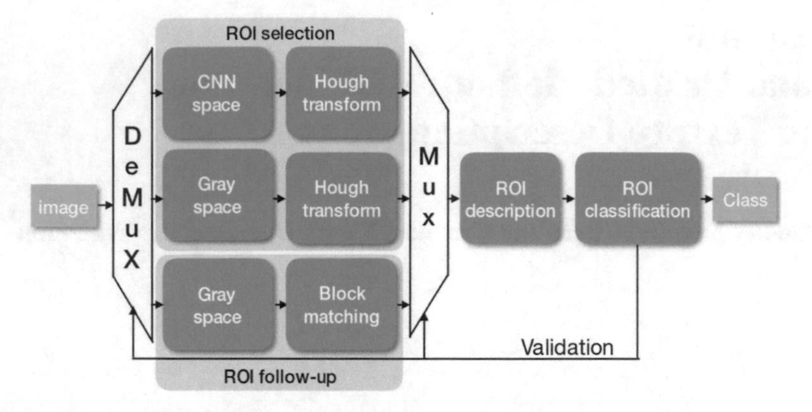

Fig. 6.1 Proposed system scheme of polyps detection

3. **ROI description stage**: in this stage, 26 texture and luminosity descriptors are extracted for each ROI. The co-occurrence matrix is used to compute them. The texture and luminosity are the important descriptors to recognize and discriminate polyps (Romain et al. 2013).
4. **ROI classification stage**: in this stage, a fuzzy forest is used to classify each ROI. An ROI containing a polyp is classified as $class1$, if not it is classified as $class0$. If any previous ROI was validated as $class1$ in the last image, we restart from stage 2, otherwise, we continue with stage 1 for the next image.

With this method, we can follow an ROI containing a polyp once it is detected. This strategy reduces the number of ROI processed per image and the number of false positives. The fuzzy forest is created with specialized fuzzy trees that recognized a particular type of polyp; this approach robustifies the classification.

In the next sections, we describe each stage of our method.

6.2 ROI Selection Stage

In this stage, we use two color spaces: a brightness model and a color model.

1. the brightness model allows an efficient texture analysis. To obtain the brightness model, the well-known formulae is applied to the RGB image $image_{out} = 0.587 * image_{in-green} + 0.299 * image_{in-red} + 0.114 * image_{in-blue}$ (B. S. B. service (television) 2011). The resulting image, $image_{out}$, is filtered by a gaussian filter to remove the noise. This model preserves the texture information and provides a good degree of integrability inside an SoC.
2. the color model enables the use of color information for image analysis. Three convolutional kernels are applied to the RGB image, one kernel by channel, and a sum, with a normalization, of the three filtered images is made, see Fig. 6.2. This

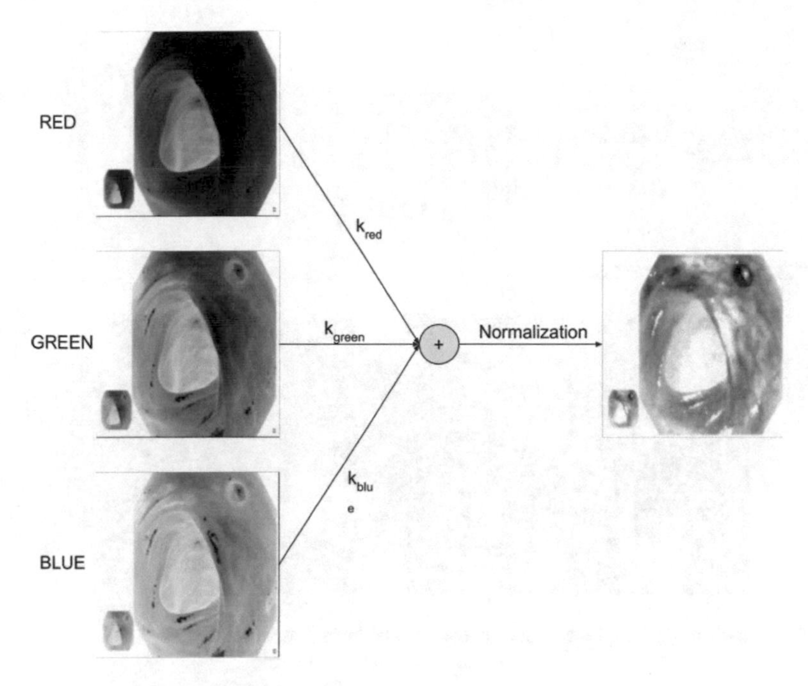

Fig. 6.2 Convolutional kernel model

model is very effective to locate a certain type of polyps and has a high degree of integrability.

On the two images from the two models, a Canny filter is applied as an edge detector (Canny 1986). Then Hough transform is used on both images to detect ellipses, each region containing an ellipse becomes an ROI.

Hough transform processing is integrable in real time in a system on chip (Tagzout et al. 2001; Orlando et al. 2018) and it is efficient processing to detect ellipse (Tagzout et al. 2001; Chen et al. 2012).

6.2.1 The Convolutional Kernels

To obtain the convolutional kernels, first a Convolutional Neural Network (CNN), the GoogleNet (Szegedy et al. 2015), is trained to classify images from colonoscopies in two classes: image containing at least one polyp and image without polyp. The architecture of this CNN is shown in Fig. 6.3.

GoogleNet implements the InceptionV3 model proposed by Google (Szegedy et al. 2015). This CNN was the winner of the 2014 ILSVRC Contest with less number of synapses and neurons in comparison with Alexnet, VGGnet, Lenet, or Resnet.

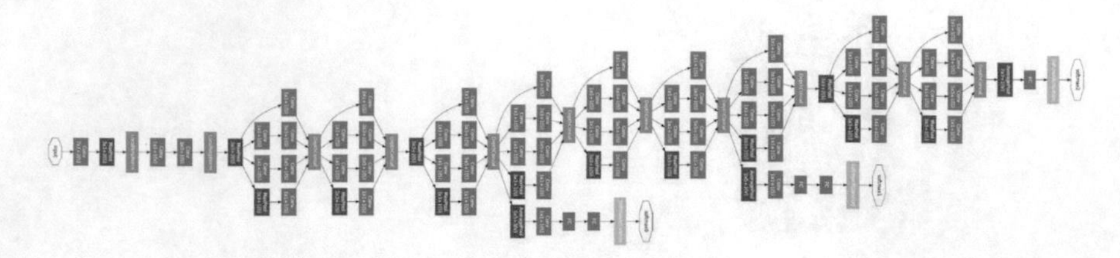

Fig. 6.3 The Googlenet CNN

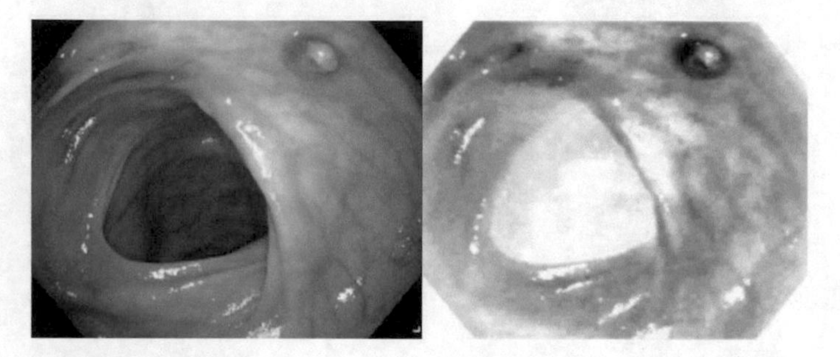

Fig. 6.4 Input image and the output of convolutional kernel number 13

We adapt its last layer, the fully connected layer, with a structure with two outputs dedicated to determining the presence of a polyp in an image.

To train this CNN, we use a 11952 images database divided into 10023 images with polyp and 1929 images without polyp. These images are issued from 18 videos of endoscopic examinations of Hospital Clinic, Barcelona, Spain. This dataset was used as train dataset for EndoVisSub2017-GIANA contest (Bernal et al. 2018). Each image is associated with a ground-truth: a binary-image that indicates the position of the polyp in the image.

We use 70% of the data to train the CNN and the remaining 30% to test this performance. The result show an accuracy of more than 98%. Although we have achieved very good accuracy, it is impossible to embed this convolutional neural network with four million parameters into a capsule.

We use then this CNN, not to integrate it inside a capsule, but to identify the good kernels to extract the useful information from a color image.

To do so, our method is to realize a visual analysis of each feature map, feature map by feature map, to identify kernels that made processing suitable to identify a polyp. For example, in Fig. 6.4, after the processing by a specific convolutional kernel, we clearly see that the area where the polyp is located has been darkened. This means that this convolutional kernel could be effective to help in the process to detect polyps.

With the visual analysis, we have identified three convolutional kernels that are

$$k_{red} = \begin{bmatrix} 0.08919 & 0.17597 & 0.14030 \\ 0.17235 & 0.28923 & 0.17626 \\ 0.13088 & 0.20982 & 0.18990 \end{bmatrix} \tag{6.1}$$

$$k_{green} = \begin{bmatrix} -0.01763 & 0.01118 & -0.04105 \\ 0.01724 & 0.05383 & -0.03952 \\ -0.04559 & -0.02233 & -0.01358 \end{bmatrix} \tag{6.2}$$

$$k_{blue} = \begin{bmatrix} -0.12489 & -0.17314 & -0.10103 \\ -0.15373 & -0.27334 & -0.20675 \\ -0.12675 & -0.22742 & -0.14564 \end{bmatrix} \tag{6.3}$$

6.3 ROI Follow-Up Stage

In the follow-up stage, prior to following an ROI validated as $class1$ in a previous image, we convert each image RGB model into a brightness model.

The motion estimation method used is the block matching algorithm. The principle is to measure the similarity between two blocks, one in the previous image I_{n-1} and the other in the current image I_n.

To do so an ROI validated as $class1$ in I_{n-1} is considered as a block $B_{p,q}$ of size $P * Q$. We note the pixel values of the block $B_{p,q}$ in the image I_{n-1}: $I_{n-1}(B_{p,q})$. $I_{n-1}(B_{p,q})$ is defined as

$$\begin{aligned} I_{n-1}(B_{p,q}) = [I_{n-1}(p, q), \ldots, I_{n-1}(p + P - 1, q), \ldots, \\ I_{n-1}(p + P - 1, q + Q - 1)] \end{aligned} \tag{6.4}$$

If the block $I_{n-1}(B_{p,q})$ is displaced from its initial position (p, q) to a new position $(p - i, q - j)$ by a motion vector $\overrightarrow{V} = (i, j)$, we obtain a new block $I_n(B_{p-i,q-j})$. To estimate if this displacement is probable, a similarity measure between $I_{n-1}(B_{p,q})$ and $I_n(B_{p-i,q-j})$ is computed using the SAD, Sum of Absolute Difference, metric.

$$SAD_{ij} = \sum_{\forall p,q \in [P*Q]} |I_{n-1}(B_{p,q}) - I_n(B_{p-i,q-j})| \tag{6.5}$$

Eight candidate motion vectors are used for each ROI validated as $class1$, as it is visible in Fig. 6.5. Between these eight motion vectors, we select the motion vector where SAD_{ij} is minimum as the probable $\overrightarrow{V} = (i, j)$. The resulting block $I_n(B_{p-i,q-j})$ becomes a ROI.

With this technique, we follow the ROI selected and classified $class1$ in the image I_{n-1}. Furthermore, we can also increase the $depth$ of the motion estimation to follow the ROI selected and classified $class1$ in the images $I_{n-1}, I_{n-2}, \ldots, I_{n-Depth}$. By default we use $Depth = 2$.

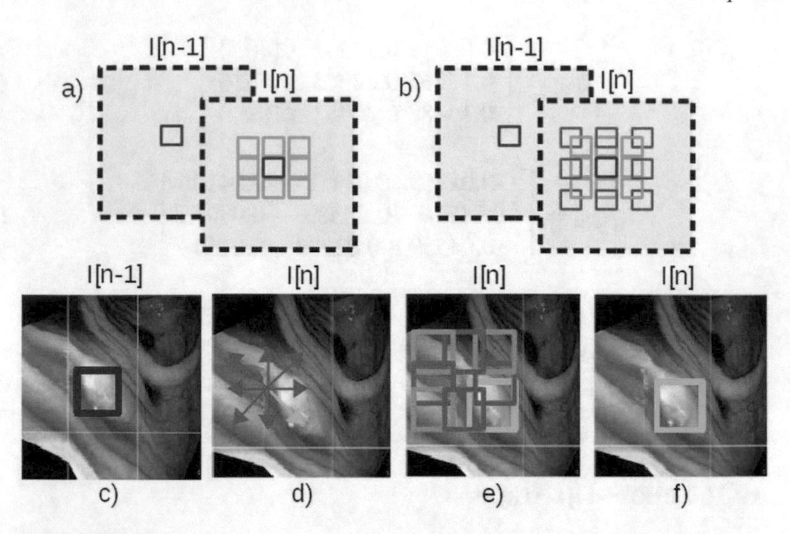

Fig. 6.5 **a** Block matching with 1 neighborhood. **b** Block matching with 2 neighborhoods. **c** ROI validated in the image I_{n-1}. **d** 8 candidate motion vectors. **e** 8 candidate blocks displaced by the candidate motion vectors. **f** Candidate block having the lowest intensity standard variation SAD_{ij}

6.4 ROI Description Stage

Each selected ROI is described by 26 texture and luminosity descriptors extracted calculating by the co-occurrence matrix (Romain et al. 2013) and the brightness histogram. Among the descriptors, we extracted the texture descriptors proposed by Haralick et al. (1973); there are autocorrelation, contrast, correlation, dissimilarity, entropy, homogeneity, maximum probability, variance, sum average, Kurtosis, and skewness.

6.5 ROI Classification Stage

In this stage, fuzzy trees and fuzzy forests are used.

6.5.1 Fuzzy Trees

This inductive recognition algorithm consists of two parts: learning phase and classification phase. In learning phase, fuzzy trees, composed of membership functions $\mu_{(x)}$, nodes, arcs v_x, and leaves $\mu_{mC_{c_k}}$, are constructed from a training dataset. In classification phase fuzzy trees classify the ROI that belongs to the class which has the highest degree of membership; there are two classes: "1" stand for ROI containing a polyp and "0" stand for ROI not containing a polyp. We aggregate one binary classification method called Classical Modus Ponem and one fuzzy classification method called Generalized Modus Ponem.

6.5.1.1 Database and Learning Phase

We used a set of 18 video-colonoscopies, in total 9894 images in which 8010 contain a polyp validated. In these videos, there is a maximum of one polyp per video and several images of the same polyp per video. These videos are issued from endoscopic examinations of Hospital Clinic, Barcelona, Spain. This dataset was used as train dataset for EndoVisSub2017-GIANA contest (Bernal et al. 2018).

From the 18 video-colonoscopies, we have obtained a dataset composed by 560388 ROI of which 228549 ROI contain a polyp $class1$. After that we have built 80 learning datasets composed by 6000 ROI where 50% belong to $class1$. In total, 80 fuzzy trees Φ are constructed from these learning datasets.

6.5.1.2 Classification Phase

To use fuzzy trees Φ to classify an observed object $\varepsilon_i\{w_1, w_2, \ldots, w_{26}\}$, we aggregate two different classification, a binary classification using the method de classical Modus Ponem and a fuzzy classification using the method of generalized Modus Ponem described below (Marsala 1998).

1. First, we calculate a satisfiability degree $Fded_{m(c_k)}$ for each class $c_k = \{0, 1\}$ and for each rule m. We calculate this using the triangular norm operator $\top$, the observed values $w_{m(j)}$ and the membership function $\mu_{j(w_{m(j)})}$ of each attribute J of the rule m multiplied by a factor called as conditional probability of Zadeh $\mu_{mC_{c_k}} = P^*(c_k/(v_{m(1)}, v_{m(2)}, \ldots, v_{m(j)}))$.

$$Fded_{m(1)} = \top_{j=1,\ldots,J}\mu_{j(w_{m(j)})} * \mu_{mC_1} \tag{6.6}$$

$$Fded_{m(0)} = \top_{j=1,\ldots,J}\mu_{j(w_{m(j)})} * \mu_{mC_0} \tag{6.7}$$

2. Finally, we calculate a new membership degree μ_{c_k} aggregating all the satisfiability degrees of each rule m using the triangular conorm operator $\perp$.

$$\mu_{polyp} = \perp_{m=1,2,\ldots,M} Fded_{m(1)} \tag{6.8}$$

$$\mu_{n\_polyp} = \perp_{m=1,2,\ldots,M} Fded_{m(0)} \tag{6.9}$$

We use the Zadeh operators to calculate triangular norm $\top_{(x,y)} = min(x, y)$ and conorm $\bot_{(x,y)} = max(x, y)$.

In the case of Classical Modus Ponem, the output is binary and the fuzzy tree is treated as a binary tree, to cross from one node to another node a comparison between the observed values $w_{m(j)}$ and the arcs or break points $v_{m(j)}$ is done for each attribute j of the rule m.

6.5.2 *Fuzzy Forest*

In order to enhance the classification rate, we construct a fuzzy forest as a combination of n fuzzy trees. We calculate a new membership degree, we aggregate the degrees of membership of the n fuzzy trees $\forall_{i=1,2,\ldots,n}\{\mu_{polyp(\Phi_i)}, \mu_{n\_polyp(\Phi_i)}\}$, this criterion is called triangular conorm "$\bot$":

$$\Upsilon_{polyp} = \bot_{i=1,2,\ldots,n}\{\mu_{polyp(\Phi_i)}\} \tag{6.10}$$

$$\Upsilon_{n\_polyp} = \bot_{i=1,2,\ldots,n}\{\mu_{n\_polyp(\Phi_i)}\} \tag{6.11}$$

In our case, for the binary classification, we propose a majority vote how triangular conorm criterion, for fuzzy classification we use the triangular criterion chosen in Sect. 6.5.1.2.

Finally, the ROI is classified as $class1$ only if both binary and fuzzy method classify the ROI as $class1$; in this case, the confidence value is the membership degree given by the fuzzy classification.

We consider that the image contains a polyp when at least 1 ROI in the image is classified as $class1$. For the (x, y) coordinates of polyp location, we give the center of the ROI detected.

6.6 Results

Figure 6.6 shows results obtained using the proposed methodology.

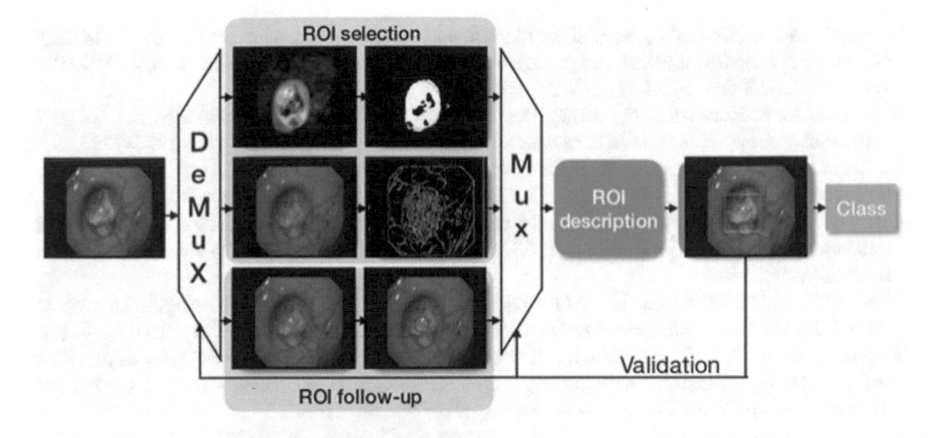

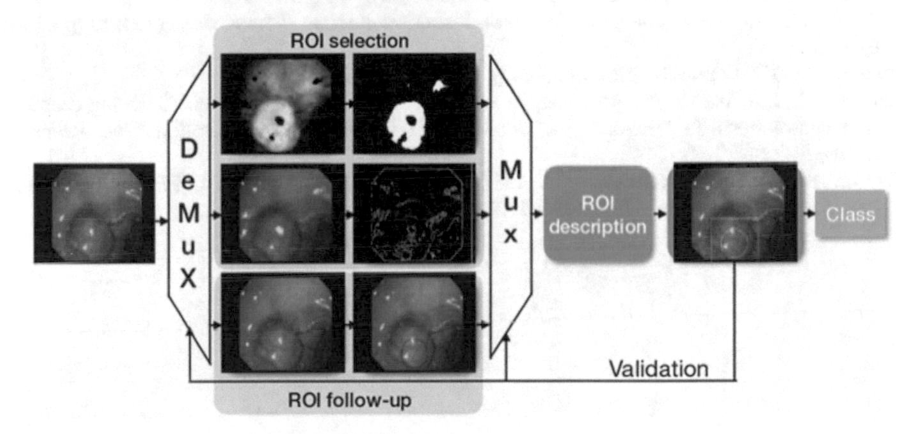

Fig. 6.6 Example of results obtained with the proposed methodology

References

Bernal, J., Histace, A., Masana, M., Angermann, Q., Sánchez-Montes, C., Rodriguez, C., et al. (2018). Polyp detection benchmark in colonoscopy videos using GTCreator: A novel fully configurable tool for easy and fast annotation of image databases. In *Proceedings of 32nd CARS Conference*.

B. S. B. service (television). (2011). Recommendation ITU-R BT.601-7 (03/2011) - Studio encoding parameters of digital television for standard 4:3 and wide-screen 16:9 aspect ratios. International Telecommunication Union.

Canny, J. (1986). A computational approach to edge detection. *IEEE Transactions on Pattern Analysis and Machine Intelligence*, *PAMI-8*, 679–698.

Chen, Z.-H., Su, A. W., & Sun, M.-T. (2012). Resource-efficient FPGA architecture and implementation of Hough transform. *IEEE Transactions on Very Large Scale Integration (VLSI) Systems*, *20*(8), 1419–1428.

Haralick, R. M., Shanmugam, K., & Dinstein, I. (1973). Textural features for image classification. *IEEE Transactions on Systems, Man, and Cybernetics*, *SMC-3*, 610–621.

Karargyris, A., & Bourbakis, N. (2009). Identification of polyps in wireless capsule endoscopy videos using Log Gabor filters. In *Life Science Systems and Applications Workshop, 2009. LiSSA 2009. IEEE/NIH* (pp. 143–147). IEEE.

Karargyris, A., & Bourbakis, N. (2011). Detection of small bowel polyps and ulcers in wireless capsule endoscopy videos. *IEEE Transactions on Biomedical Engineering*, *58*, 2777–2786.

Mamonov, A. V., Figueiredo, I. N., Figueiredo, P. N., & Tsai, Y.-H. R. (2014). Automated polyp detection in colon capsule endoscopy. *IEEE Transactions on Medical Imaging*, *33*(7), 1488–1502.

Marsala, C. (1998). Apprentissage inductif en présence de données imprécises: construction et utilisation d'arbres de décision flous, P. 232. (Doctoral dissertation, Paris 6). http://www.theses.fr/1998PA066227.

Orlando, C., Andrea, P., Xavier, D., & Granado, B. (2017). Polyps recognition using fuzzy trees. In *2017 IEEE EMBS International Conference on Biomedical Health Informatics (BHI)* (pp. 9–12).

Orlando, C., Andrea, P., Christophel, M., Xavier, D., & Granado, B. (2018). FPGA-based real time embedded Hough transform architecture for circles detection. In *2018 Conference on Design and Architectures for Signal and Image Processing (DASIP)* (pp. 31–36).

Romain, O., Histace, A., Silva, J., Ayoub, J., Granado, B., Pinna, A., et al. (2013). Towards a multimodal wireless video capsule for detection of colonic polyps as prevention of colorectal cancer. In *2013 IEEE 13th International Conference on Bioinformatics and Bioengineering (BIBE)* (pp. 1–6). IEEE.

Swain, P. (2003). Wireless capsule endoscopy. *Gut*, *52*, iv48–iv50.

Szegedy, C., Liu, W., Jia, Y., Sermanet, P., Reed, S., Anguelov, D., et al. (2015). Going deeper with convolutions. In *Proceedings of the IEEE Conference on Computer Vision and Pattern Recognition* (pp. 1–9).

Tagzout, S., Achour, K., & Djekoune, O. (2001). Hough transform algorithm for FPGA implementation. *Signal Processing*, *81*(6), 1295–1301.

Chapter 7
AECNN: Adversarial and Enhanced Convolutional Neural Networks

Saeed Izadi and Ghassan Hamarneh

7.1 Introduction

The proposed method for segmenting gastrointestinal polyps from colonoscopy images uses an adversarial and enhanced convolutional neural networks (AECNN). As the number of training images is small, the core of AECNN relies on fine-tuning an existing deep CNN model (ResNet152). AECNN's enhanced convolutions incorporate both dense upsampling, which learns to upsample the low-resolution feature maps into pixel-level segmentation masks, as well as hybrid dilation, which improves the dilated convolution by using different dilation rates for different layers. AECNN further boosts the performance of its segmenter by incorporating a discriminator competing with the segmenter, where both are trained through a generative adversarial network formulation.

7.2 Methodology

The architecture of this method is shown in Fig. 7.1. Given the limited number of training images, we fine-tune a fully convolutional version of the ResNet152 model (He et al. 2016), pre-trained on ImageNet (Russakovsky et al. 2015), for segmenting the gastrointestinal polyps in colonoscopy images. To tackle the problem of low-resolution feature maps caused by max-pooling operations, we utilize the method of Wang et al. (2017) to incorporate a dense upsampling convolution (DUC) module, as the final component of the network, which learns to upsample the low-resolution

S. Izadi (✉) · G. Hamarneh
School of Computing Science, Simon Fraser University, Burnaby, Canada
e-mail: saeedi@sfu.ca

G. Hamarneh
e-mail: hamarneh@sfu.ca

J. Bernal and A. Histace (eds.), *Computer-Aided Analysis of Gastrointestinal Videos*,
https://doi.org/10.1007/978-3-030-64340-9_7

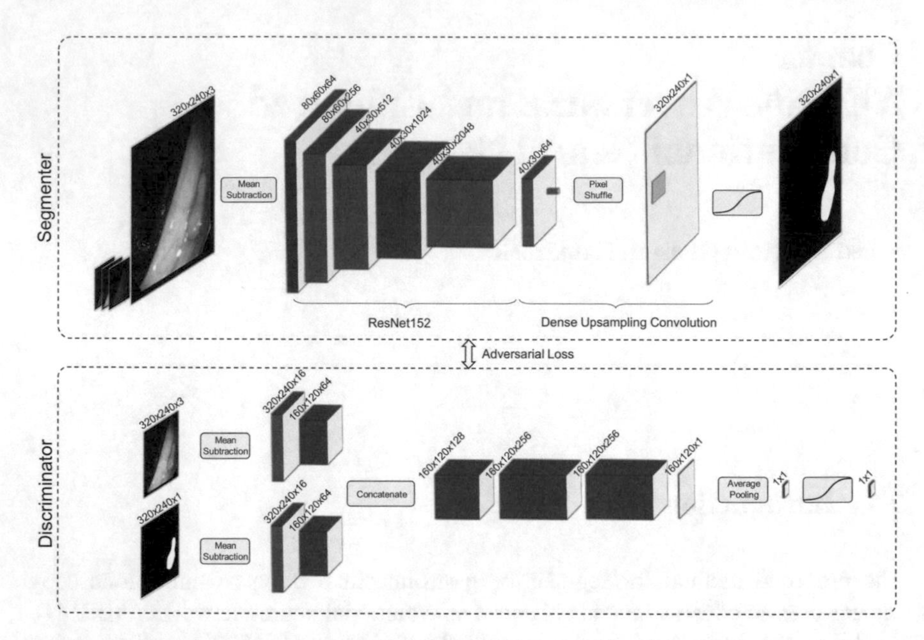

Fig. 7.1 The schematic of the proposed AECNN model for polyp segmentation. The error in the discriminator is backpropagated through the segmenter to make it produce more realistic segmentation masks

feature maps into pixel-level segmentation maps. Compared to non-learnable upsampling techniques, e.g., bilinear interpolation, the DUC technique leads to finer boundaries. We also exploit dilated convolutional operations (Yu and Koltun 2016), which enlarge the valid receptive field of our model, in order to improve the segmentation performance, especially for large polyps. Wang et al. (2017) also highlighted the "gridding effect" problem with dilated convolutions and proposed a simple yet effective solution to tackle it. Instead of using the same dilation rate after the downsampling stage, they suggested different dilation rates for each subsequent layer in a sawtooth wave-like fashion. Particularly, a number of layers are grouped together to form a "rising edge" of the wave that has an increasing dilation rate, and the next group repeats the same pattern. We also found, in our experiments, the approach of Wang et al. effective for segmenting objects with large objects.

Inspired by the works of Pan et al. (2017) and Luc et al. (2016), we further boost the performance of our model by adding a discriminator network to distinguish ground truth from generated prediction maps. Specifically, we feed the loss value of the discriminator network back to the segmenter. When the segmenter-discriminator are trained alternately, the adversarial scenario causes the two networks to compete against each other: The segmenter learns to produce prediction maps that are difficult for the discriminator to distinguish from the ground truth mask, while the discriminator attempts to correctly distinguish the true (i.e., ground truth) from the synthesized (i.e., automatically predicted) label masks (Sect. 7.3). Our qualitative experiments show that this adversarial competition leads the segmenter model to uniformly highlight the polyp regions and ignore irrelevant features in the final prediction map. As data augmentation, we inflate the training set by applying rotation, horizontal, and vertical flipping. All images are also resized to 240×320. We post-process the binarized prediction results with one iteration of morphological closing and opening operations with a 5×5 structuring element to remove any remaining isolated pixels or small holes.

7.3 Generative Adversarial Networks

Generative adversarial networks (Goodfellow et al. 2014), GANs in short, have been recently introduced as a way to train generative models in the scope of deep learning. Typically, GAN models consist of two sub-models, a generator and a discriminator which are trained jointly in an adversarial atmosphere. The generator network G receives a noise sample z from a random distribution p_z and produces a realistic sample x via capturing the data distribution p_{data}, while the discriminator D takes the generated sample x as the input and determines whether it came from the true distribution p_{true} or the one learned by G. Once trained adversarially, the generator G attempts to produce realistic data samples that fools the discriminator. Nevertheless, the discriminator's ultimate goal is to perfectly distinguish between the synthetic and real samples. Both G and D are trained alternately in a two-player training framework using the following objective function:

$$\min_G \max_D L(D, G) = \mathbb{E}_{x \sim p_{data}(x)}[\log D(x)] + \mathbb{E}_{z \sim p_z}(z)[\log(1 - D(G(z)))] \quad (7.1)$$

Conditional generative adversarial network (Mirza and Osindero 2014), CGAN for short, is a variant of GANs where the generator and/or discriminator are conditioned on some extra information. The conditioning is typically performed by exposing the information as inputs to the networks. For binary segmentation, this extra information is provided by the ground truth binary mask y as the input to the discriminative model during the training. The objective function of CGAN is as follows:

$$\min_G \max_D L(D, G) = \mathbb{E}_{x \sim p_{data}(x)}[\log D(x|y)] + \mathbb{E}_{z \sim p_z}(z)[\log(1 - D(G(z)))] \quad (7.2)$$

It is noteworthy that for image segmentation, the input of the generator z is the image to be segmented.

References

Goodfellow, I. J., Pouget-Abadie, J., Mirza, M., Xu, B., Warde-Farley, D., Ozair, S., et al. (2014). Generative adversarial networks.

He, K., Zhang, X., Ren, S., & Sun, J. (2016). Deep residual learning for image recognition. In *Proceedings of the IEEE Conference on Computer Vision and Pattern Recognition* (pp. 770–778).

Luc, P., Couprie, C., Chintala, S., & Verbeek, J. (2016). Semantic segmentation using adversarial networks. arXiv:1611.08408.

Mirza, M., & Osindero, S. (2014). Conditional generative adversarial nets. arXiv:1411.1784.

Pan, J., Canton, C., McGuinness, K., O'Connor, N. E., Torres, J., Sayrol, E., et al. (2017). SalGAN: Visual saliency prediction with adversarial networks. In *CVPR Scene Understanding Workshop (SUNw)*.

Russakovsky, O., Deng, J., Su, H., Krause, J., Satheesh, S., Ma, S., et al. (2015). ImageNet large scale visual recognition challenge. *International Journal of Computer Vision*, *115*(3), 211–252.

Wang, P., Chen, P., Yuan, Y., Liu, D., Huang, Z., Hou, X., et al. (2017). Understanding convolution for semantic segmentation. arXiv:1702.08502.

Yu, F., & Koltun, V. (2016). Multi-scale context aggregation by dilated convolutions. In *ICLR*.

Chapter 8
Dilated ResFCN and SE-Unet for Polyp Segmentation

Yunbo Guo and Bogdan J. Matuszewski

8.1 Motivation

Segmentation is one of the key enabling technologies in medical image analysis with a great variety of methods proposed (Histace et al. 2009; Zhang et al. 2010, 2013; Matuszewski et al. 2011). Methods based on deep learning, with the features learned directly from data rather than handcrafted, showed significant improvement in the quality of the segmentation including the analysis of colonoscopy images. The recent advances in fully convolutional networks and in particular the dilation convolution and squeeze-and-excitation unit have inspired the two architectures proposed in this chapter. More specifically, the first proposed network can be seen as a specific example of an encoder-decoder architecture with the multi-channel encoder providing features operating at different spatial resolution of the input image. The dilation kernels in each channel facilitate a compromise between the capacity of the network and the size of the receptive fields. The second network combines the base U-net architecture with squeeze-and-excitation units, to take better advantage of the extracted features. Overall, the key motivation behind the proposed solutions is to strike a balance between network capacity and the size of the receptive field. The objective is to use a possibly large receptive field, without significantly increasing the network capacity. This way, the network is less prone to overfitting, particularly when trained on relatively small data sets with somewhat limited dimensionality of the underlying segmentation problem.

Y. Guo · B. J. Matuszewski
Computer Vision and Machine Learning (CVML) Group, School of Engineering,
University of Central Lancashire, Preston PR1 2HE, UK
e-mail: bmatuszewski1@uclan.ac.uk

Y. Guo (✉)
Suzhou Institute of Biomedical Engineering and Technology,
China Academy of Sciences, Suzhou, China
e-mail: YBGuo1@uclan.ac.uk; guoyb@sibet.ac.c

J. Bernal and A. Histace (eds.), *Computer-Aided Analysis of Gastrointestinal Videos*,
https://doi.org/10.1007/978-3-030-64340-9_8

8.2 Introduction of the Base Structure

The fully convolutional network (FCN) architecture was the first type of end-to-end network to be successfully used for semantic image segmentation based on deep learning (Long et al. 2015). FCN can process images of any size and obtain a full-size segmentation result without the need for additional pre-processing. The structure of an FCN can be divided into two parts, an encoder and a decoder. The former is used to extract low resolution, high-level features from the input image. The latter fuses these features and converts them into low-resolution segmentation results, then restores their size by means of up-sampling and cropping layers. The loss in the backward direction is determined by processing the full-scale segmentation result and ground truth. Then, the errors are propagated to each hidden layer that needs to be trained. This method not only simplifies the steps of image segmentation, but also is more accurate than the traditional methods.

Encoder

The encoder can be any CNN whose fully connected layer has been removed. It can be one of the existing CNN architectures or a custom built one. When designing an FCN, the choice of the encoder is usually determined by the complexity of the images and the performance of the hardware, with the goal of avoiding unnecessary calculations. It should be noted that when using an FCN model, the final feature map is required to be of a certain size, otherwise, some smaller objects of interest could be missed. Therefore, the rate of down-sampling should be chosen based on the characteristics of the specific segmentation problem.

Decoder

The decoder consists of a pixel classifier, an up-sampling layer and a cropping layer. The pixel classifier is used to classify the pixels in the feature maps one by one. It is a convolutional layer rather than a fully connected layer. This is because the number of outputs of a fully connected layer is fixed, making it impossible to process images of different sizes. For general pixel classifiers, a 1×1 convolution kernel is used to fuse the feature maps and generate low-resolution segmentation results. Large convolution kernels can also be used, but additional padding is needed to ensure that the size of the feature maps is not significantly reduced.

To reduce the loss of segmentation details caused by down-sampling, feature maps of different resolutions can be extracted from convolution layers at different depths in the encoder, and corresponding pixel classifiers can then be designed separately. After that, the results can be fused through up-sampling, creating the so-called skip structure (Long et al. 2015). As the fusion method, a direct addition could be used, or build structures are stacked and fused by using a 1×1 convolution kernel. The up-sampling layer is a critical hidden layer in an FCN, and it serves as the basis for end-to-end training. The up-sampling layer is essentially a special convolutional layer controlled by a set of three parameters, namely, the size of the convolution kernel, the stride and the kernel weighs. The stride size corresponds to the scale of previous down-sampling operations. The kernel weights often are selected to correspond to bilinear interpolation, subsequently in some cases, they are adjusted during the network training. Finally, the up-sampled results are cropped to match the size of the ground truth.

The original architecture of FCN inducted three sub-architectures, namely, FCN32s, FCN16s and FCN8s (Long et al. 2015) (Fig. 8.1). In all three, VGG16 was used as an encoder. The difference in the sub-architecture is that the sizes of the skip structures are different. FCN8s performs classification after FC7, pool4 and pool3 and generates a corresponding segmentation result for each case. VGG16 contains a total of 5 down-sampling layers, and each output is reduced by a factor of 2. Therefore, the results of the last two down-sampling layers are required to be up-sampled and then merged with the result of the pool3 classifier to obtain the final segmentation result. Since the output of pool3 is only 1/8th the size of the original image, the fusion result needs to be enlarged by a factor of 8 (hence the name FCN8s). In FCN16s classifiers are included only after pool4 and FC7, and their outputs are fused. The output of pool4 is 1/16th the size of the original image, so the segmentation result needs to be enlarged by a factor of 16. FCN32s uses only the output of FC7 as the segmentation result.

One of the important concepts in the design of FCN is the receptive field, which refers to the size of the area in the input image to which each unit in the output layer corresponds. A larger receptive field allows the output to contain more global features, which helps to improve the accuracy of the segmentation results. However, reducing the stride for down-sampling to improve local spatial segmentation accuracy will make the receptive field smaller.

In the example shown in Fig. 8.2, when the pooling stride is 2 (Fig. 8.2a), the receptive field is 6 (a single output unit is connected to 6 input units). When the pooling stride becomes 1 (Fig. 8.2b), the output size is increased to 7, but only 4 input units are connected to a single output unit. In this case, there is no doubt that the output size is improved, but the amount of information contained in each output unit is reduced.

Using a larger convolution kernel can solve this problem, but it will increase the computational cost and the number of parameters to be estimated, as shown in Fig. 8.2c. To solve this problem more efficiently, the so-called dilated convolution (Yu and Koltun 2016) (also known as atrous convolution) was proposed. The underlying idea is to increase the size of the convolution kernel by adding 0s between the weights without changing the number of weights, as shown in Fig. 8.2d. The definition of the dilated convolution is given as

$$y[i] = \sum_{k=1}^{K} x[i + r \times k]w[k]$$

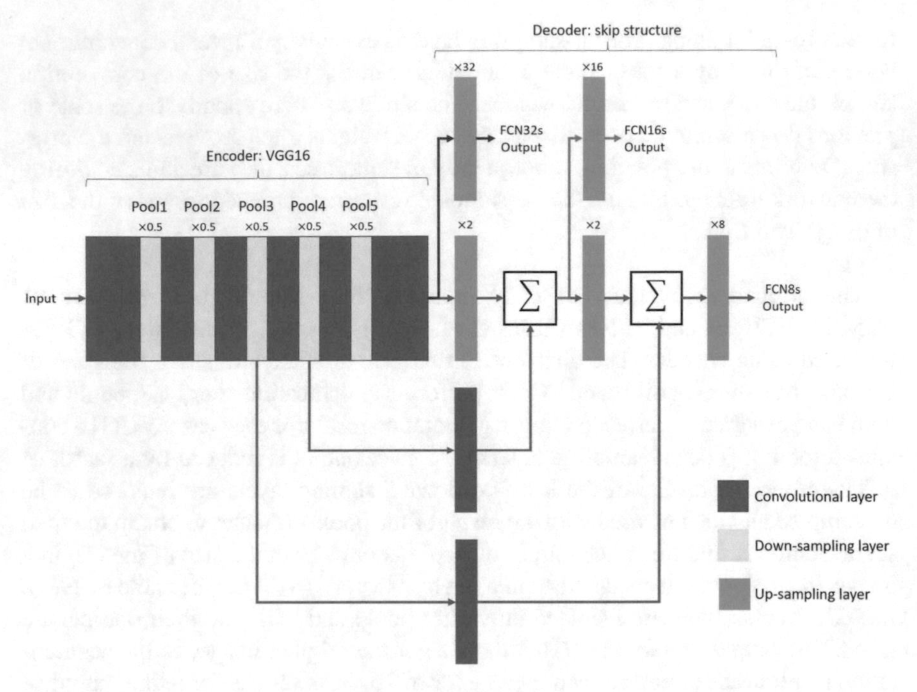

Fig. 8.1 The structure of FCN8s, FCN16s and FCN32s

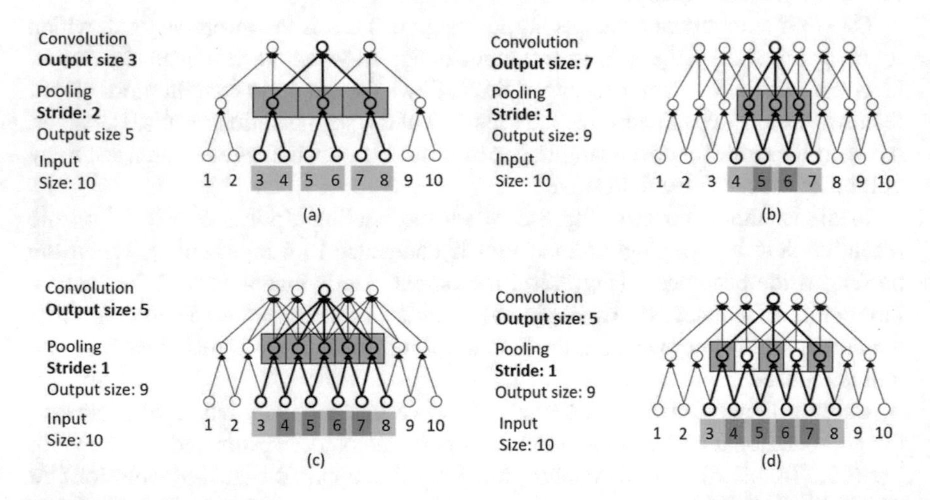

Fig. 8.2 Regular convolution (**a**)–(**c**) and atrous convolution (**d**). **a** Regular convolution, with pooling stride 2 and 1×3 kernel. **b** Regular convolution, with pooling stride 1 and 1×3 kernel. **c** Regular convolution, with pooling stride 1 and 1×5 kernel. **d** Atrous convolution, with pooling stride 1, 1×5 kernel and dilation 2; kernel size is 5 but only 3 weights are trainable

where $y[i]$ is the output, x[i] is an 1-D input signal, $w[k]$ represents the weight in a kernel. The parameter r is called dilation rate and it controls the stride between each weight in an atrous kernel.

8.3 Methodology Explanation

Based on analysis of existing machine learning and polyp image segmentation techniques, a novel hybrid deep learning segmentation method (Guo and Matuszewski 2019, 2020; Guo 2019) has been proposed for both SD and HD GIANA polyp segmentation problems. The method consists of two fully convolutional networks. The first network named "Dilated ResFCN" takes advantage of dilation convolution layers (Chen et al. 2017) to increase receptive fields, and therefore, makes the algorithm aware of various multi-scale relationships between the polyps and their surroundings. The second network "SE-Unet" is designed to segment small and flat polyps which have been missed by the Dilated ResFCN, however, overall it tends to produce more false positive pixels.

8.3.1 Dilated ResFCN

The architecture of the first proposed network, Dilated ResFCN, is shown in Fig. 8.3. This architecture is inspired by Long et al. (2015), Chen et al. (2017), and the Global Convolutional Network (Peng et al. 2017). The proposed FCN consists of three subnetworks performing specific tasks: feature extraction, multi-resolution classification and fusion. The feature extraction sub-network is based on the ResNet-50 model (He et al. 2016).

The classification sub-network consists of four parallel paths. Each such path includes a dilation convolutional layer, which is used to increase the receptive field without increasing computational complexity. The larger receptive fields are needed to access contextual information about polyp neighbourhood areas. The dilation rate is determined by the number of active kernel weights (Guo and Matuszewski 2020). The dilation rates for sub-nets connected to Res5-Res2 are 2, 4, 8, 16 and the corresponding kernel sizes are 5, 9, 17 and 33. The fusion sub-network corresponds to the deconvolution layers of the FCN model. The segmentation results from each classification sub-network are up-sampled and fused by a bilinear interpolation.

The feature extraction sub-network weights are initialized by a publicly available ResNet-50 (Deep residual networks 2017). The convolutional layers in the four parallel classification paths are initialized by the Xavier method (Glorot and Bengio 2010).

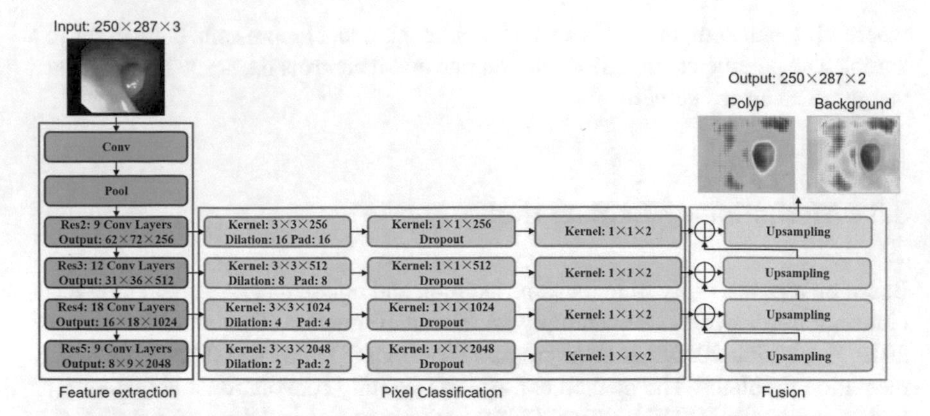

Fig. 8.3 Dilated ResFCN polyp segmentation network, with the feature extraction sub-network (in blue) based on the ResNet, the multi-resolution classification sub-network (in yellow) based on the dilated convolution, and the fusion sub-network (in green) using bilinear interpolation

8.3.2 SE-Unet

The Dilated ResFCN focuses on learning features using a larger receptive field. However, smaller polyps may be ignored by networks with a large receptive field, this is because smaller polyps may not excite lower resolution feature maps strongly enough. To solve this problem, the SE-Unet network has been proposed. It has been designed specifically for the detection and segmentation of small polyps missed by the Dilated ResFCN network.

The SE-Unet, shown in Fig. 8.4, is based on the classic U-net architecture (Ronneberger et al. 2015). In the encoder, the original architecture of U-net is replaced by the VGG16 network (Simonyan and Zisserman 2015), and a modified atrous spatial pyramid pooling (ASPP) module (Chen et al. 2017). The ASPP module has four kernels, with respective sizes of 1×1, 3×3, 5×5, 7×7. The last two are dilated kernels, with corresponding dilation rates of 2 and 4. These two modifications have the purpose of improving the performance of image feature extraction. The decoder can be regarded as a mirrored VGG16 network where the down-sampling layers are replaced by up-sampling layers. The original U-net fuses different level feature maps after each up-sampling layer to provide more features to the pixel level classifier. In SE-Unet, this is further reinforced with the squeeze-and-excitation (SE) module (Hu et al. 2018) added between the up-sampling and fusion layer. The SE module aims to assign higher weights to the high importance features and lower weights to minor importance features and therefore the network is expected to focus more on important features in the decoder. The parameter “r” in the SE module is set to 16. The SE-Unet training consists of two stages. In the first stage, the SE modules are removed from SE-Unet. In the second stage, the SE modules are added and the whole network is re-trained. Both Dilated ResFCN and SE-Unet are trained using the Adam algorithm.

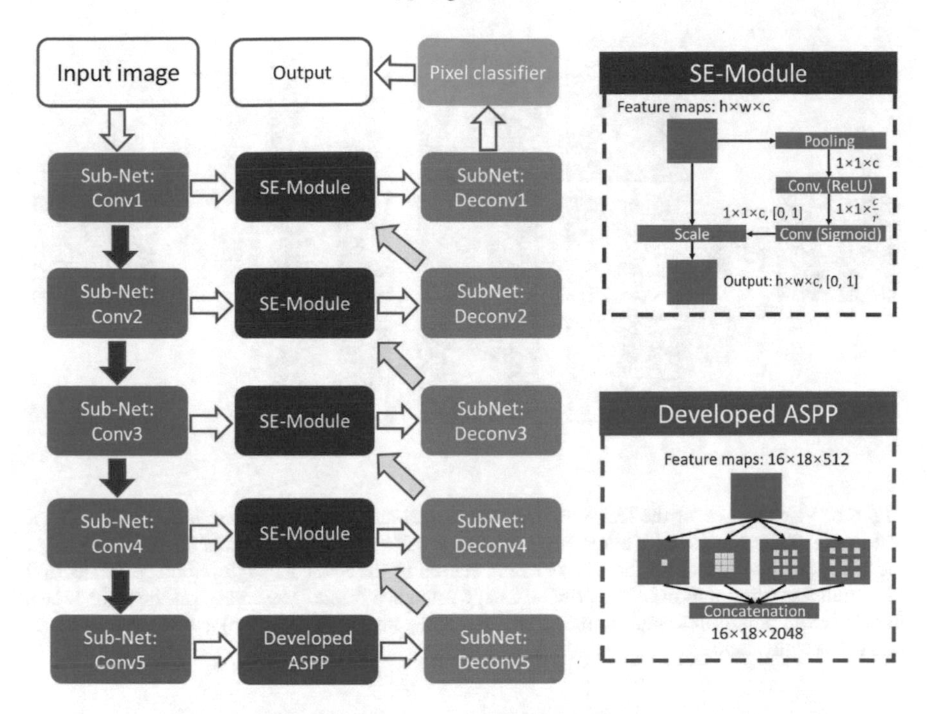

Fig. 8.4 SE-Unet polyp segmentation network with SE-module to introduce attention gating to better utilize information in the computed feature maps and atrous spatial pyramid pooling (ASPP) to effectively control receptive filed

8.3.3 Training-Time Data Augmentation

One of the key advantages of deep learning is that features are learned directly from data rather than been designed/handcrafted. Therefore, in many cases, these features inherently better represent complex data. However, for this to work, the training data should adequately represent data variabilities, including size, pose, shape, texture, colour, etc. From that perspective, the training data available for the GIANA polyp segmentation challenge was rather small. Therefore, available data were heavily augmented with random rotation, translation, scale changes as well as colour and contrast jitter. In total, after augmentation, the training dataset consisted of more than 90,000 images.

8.3.4 Test-Time Data Augmentation

Since the convolutional neural networks are not inherently rotation invariant, a possible option to improve segmentation results is to perform the data augmentation during the test time (Simonyan and Zisserman 2015). For this, rotated versions of the origi-

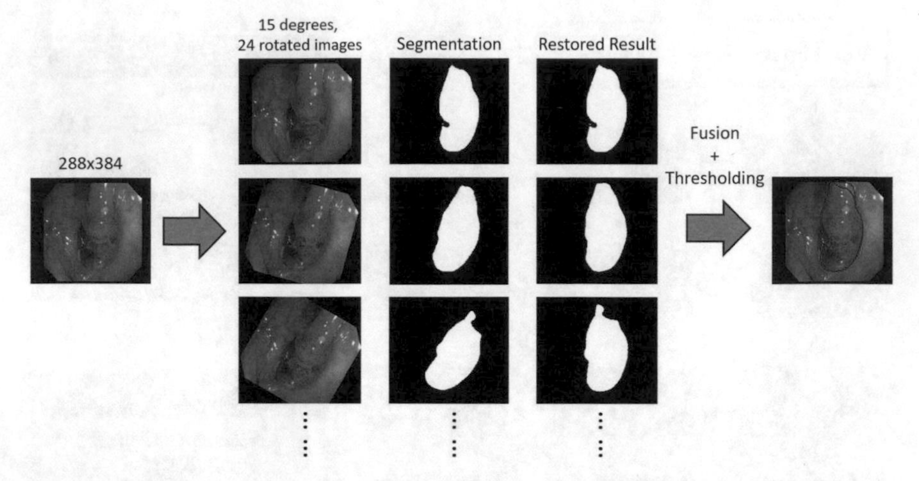

Fig. 8.5 Visualization of the test-time data augmentation. The image on the left shows an input test image. Images in the middle represent rotated, in 15° intervals, versions of the original image; the corresponding results of the binary segmentation in the rotated image reference frame; and the results after restoration to the original image reference frame. The image on the right shows final segmentation results, superimposed on the original image, with (in red) and without (in blue) test-time augmentation

nal test image are also presented to the network and the corresponding outputs, after restoring to the original image reference frame, are averaged to take advantage of the network generalization capabilities. The adopted test-time augmentation process is explained in Fig. 8.5. The implemented augmentation uses 24 images derived from the original test image rotated in 15° intervals.

8.4 Example of Results

This section presents validation results of the proposed methods using GIANA SD training images, with a standard 4-fold cross-validation scheme. Frames extracted from the same video are always in the same validation sub-set, i.e. they are not used for training and validation at the same time. The three main configurations have been tested: Dilated ResFCN, SE-Unet and the hybrid method. The hybrid method uses Dilated ResFCN as the base network and switches to the SE-Unet when the base network does not detect any polyps. These three architectures have been compared against the FCN8s and simplified version of the Dilated ResFCN, called here ResFCN. The ResFCN has the same architecture like the one shown in Fig. 8.3, but without the dilation kernels. This network has been included to demonstrate the significance of the dilation kernels on the segmentation performance.

Figure 8.6 shows a sample of segmentation results for typical small, medium and large polyps. The polyp occurrence confidence maps show that FCN8s can

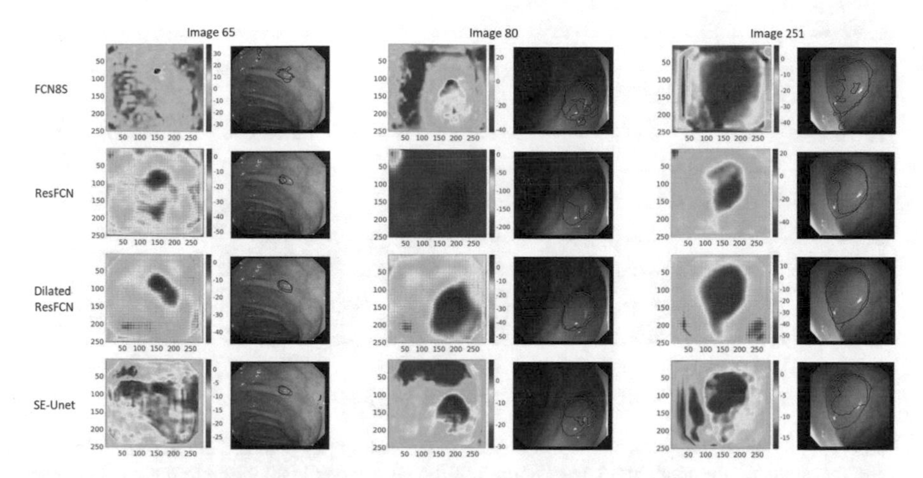

Fig. 8.6 Typical results obtained for the SD images using FCN8s, ResFCN, Dilated ResFCN and SE-Unet networks (Guo 2019). For each image: the left column shows the polyp occurrence confidence maps with the red colour representing the high confidence and blue colour representing the low confidence of a polyp presence; the right column shows the original images with superimposed red and blue contours representing the ground truth and segmentation results, respectively

Table 8.1 Mean Dice index obtained on 4-fold validation data using Dilated ResFCN network

	Dice		Precision		Recall		Hausdorff	
	Mean	Std	Mean	Std	Mean	Std	Mean	Std
FCN8s	0.63	0.11	0.68	0.10	0.65	0.12	193	76
ResFCN	0.71	0.08	0.75	0.07	0.74	0.09	201	110
Dilated ResFCN	0.79	0.08	0.81	0.07	0.81	0.09	54	21
SE-Unet	0.70	0.06	0.75	0.04	0.71	0.06	109	28
Hybrid	0.80	0.06	0.84	0.06	0.82	0.07	61	21

determine the approximate position of a polyp, but it generates a large number of false positives and false negatives with diffused network response and irregular shape of the segmented polyps. For the large polyp, FCN8s generate many strong responses outside of the polyp. For the Dilated ResFCN, the confidence maps are more accurate than those of the other methods with a clear boundary defining polyp edges.

Table 8.1 presents the corresponding results for the Dice Index, Precision, Recall and the Hausdorff distance metrics. It can be seen that overall all best results are provided by the hybrid method closely followed by the Dilated ResFCN, indeed the latter outperforms the former with respect to the Hausdorff distance.

Figure 8.7 shows a more detailed representation of the mean Dice index results achieved by the tested methods. For each method, the results are shown as histograms of a number of polyps calculated as a function of the Dice index. It can be observed that Dilated ResFCN segments the largest number of polyps within the top Dice index

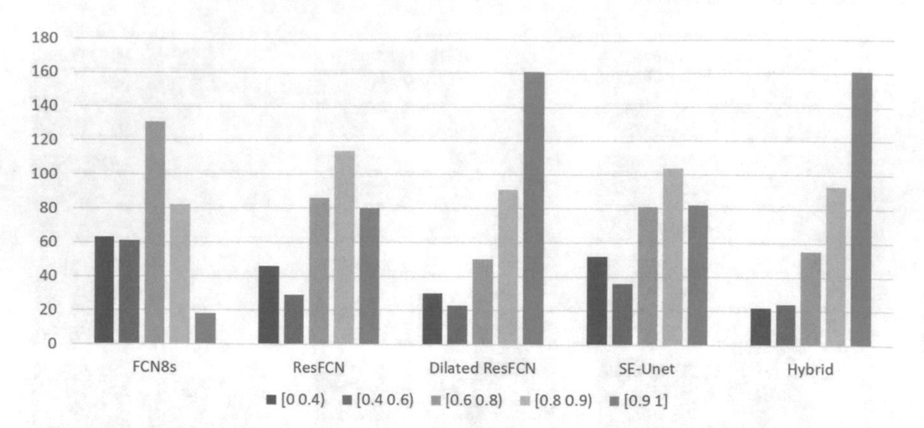

Fig. 8.7 Number of polyps as a function of Dice index histograms obtained on validation data for different segmentation methods. The definition of the Dice index histogram bin intervals is given below the graph

range (i.e. with the Dice index between 0.9 and 1). The Hybrid method produces very similar results within the top range, but improving (reducing the number of polyps) within the bottom range (i.e. with the Dice index between 0 and 0.4), due to improvement in segmentation of small polyps.

References

Chen, L.-C., Papandreou, G., Kokkinos, I., Murphy, K., & Yuille, A. L. (2017). DeepLab: Semantic image segmentation with deep convolutional nets, atrous convolution, and fully connected CRFs. *IEEE Transactions on Pattern Analysis and Machine Intelligence, 40*(4), 834–848.

Deep residual networks. https://github.com/KaimingHe/deep-residual-networks. Retrieved 03 August 2017.

Glorot, X., & Bengio, Y. (2010). Understanding the difficulty of training deep feedforward neural networks. In *Proceedings of the Thirteenth International Conference on Artificial Intelligence and Statistics* (pp. 249–256).

Guo, Y., & Matuszewski, B. J. (2020). Polyp segmentation with fully convolutional deep dilation neural network. In Zheng, Y., Williams, B., Chen, K. (Eds.) *Medical Image Understanding and Analysis. MIUA* (2019). Communications in Computer and Information Science, vol 1065. Springer, Cham

Guo, Y. B. (2019). *Polyp segmentation in colonoscopy images with convolutional neural networks*. Ph.D. thesis, University of Central Lancashire.

Guo, Y. B., & Matuszewski, B. (2019). GIANA polyp segmentation with fully convolutional dilation neural networks. In *Proceedings of the 14th International Joint Conference on Computer Vision, Imaging and Computer Graphics Theory and Applications* (pp. 632–641). SCITEPRESS-Science and Technology Publications.

He, K., Zhang, X., Ren, S., & Sun, J. (2016). Deep residual learning for image recognition. In *Proceedings of the IEEE Conference on Computer Vision and Pattern Recognition* (pp. 770–778).

Histace, A., Matuszewski, B. J., & Zhang, Y. (2009). Segmentation of myocardial boundaries in tagged cardiac MRI using active contours: A gradient-based approach integrating texture analysis. *International Journal of Biomedical Imaging*, *2009*, 983794:1–983794:8.

Hu, J., Shen, L., & Sun, G. (2018). Squeeze-and-excitation networks. In *Proceedings of the IEEE Conference on Computer Vision and Pattern Recognition* (pp. 7132–7141).

Long, J., Shelhamer, E., & Darrell, T. (2015). Fully convolutional networks for semantic segmentation. In *Proceedings of the IEEE Conference on Computer Vision and Pattern Recognition* (pp. 3431–3440).

Matuszewski, B. J., Murphy, M. F., Burton, D. R., Marchant, T. E., Moore, C. J., Histace, A., et al. (2011). Segmentation of cellular structures in actin tagged fluorescence confocal microscopy images. In *2011 18th IEEE International Conference on Image Processing* (pp. 3081–3084).

Peng, C., Zhang, X., Yu, G., Luo, G., & Sun, J. (2017). Large kernel matters–improve semantic segmentation by global convolutional network. In *IEEE Conference on Computer Vision and Pattern Recognition (CVPR)*, Honolulu, HI, USA (pp. 1743–1751). IEEE.

Ronneberger, O., Fischer, P., & Brox, T. (2015). U-Net: Convolutional networks for biomedical image segmentation. In *International Conference on Medical Image Computing and Computer-Assisted Intervention* (pp. 234–241). Springer.

Simonyan, K., & Zisserman, A. (2015). Very deep convolutional networks for large-scale image recognition. In *3rd International Conference on Learning Representations, (ICLR)*, San Diego, CA, USA. May 7–9arXiv:1409.1556.

Yu, F., & Koltun, V. (2016). Multi-scale context aggregation by dilated convolutions. In /textit4th International Conference on Learning Representations, (ICLR), San Juan, Puerto Rico. May 2–4. arXiv:1511.07122.

Zhang, Y., Matuszewski, B. J., Histace, A., Precioso, F., Kilgallon, J., & Moore, C. (2010). Boundary delineation in prostate imaging using active contour segmentation method with interactively defined object regions. In *International Workshop on Prostate Cancer Imaging* (pp. 131–142). Springer.

Zhang, Y., Matuszewski, B. J., Histace, A., & Precioso, F. (2013). Statistical model of shape moments with active contour evolution for shape detection and segmentation. *Journal of Mathematical Imaging and Vision, 47*(1–2), 35–47.

Chapter 9
Multi-encoder Decoder Network for Polyp Detection

Ahmed Mohammed and Marius Pedersen

9.1 Motivation

A typical approach to polyp detection algorithm using deep learning involves either training a model from scratch or fine-tuning learned weights through transfer learning. However, in this work, we propose a deep learning architecture that exploits fine-tuning and random initialization of weights in a multi-encoder with a single decoder network architecture. The architecture follows encode-decoder design strategy as it has been shown in the literature to give a state-of-the-art semantic image segmentation result for medical applications (Ronneberger et al. 2015). The architecture is novel in that randomly initialized and fine tuned features are fused at each stage of the encoder network and concatenated with the decoder of a similar stage. Moreover, the proposed encoder specific learning rate to train the architecture allows for gradual fine-tuning of the pretrained and randomly initialized weights. A generalized multi-encoder decoder approach is shown in Fig. 9.1.

9.2 Y-Net for Polyp Detection

This work is based on Mohammed et al. (2018, 2019)[1] using two encoders. The approach focuses on using the pretrained model features optimally by slow fine-tuning the pretrained network and aggressive learning on the second encoder for a better generalization on the test set. The framework consists of two fully convolution encoder networks which are connected to a single decoder network that matches the encoder network resolution at each down-sampling operation. The main goal

[1] Source code supporting this publication is available at https://ahme0307.github.io/.

A. Mohammed (✉) · M. Pedersen
Norwegian University of Science and Technology, 2815 Gjøvik, Norway
e-mail: mohammed.kedir@ntnu.no

J. Bernal and A. Histace (eds.), *Computer-Aided Analysis of Gastrointestinal Videos*,
https://doi.org/10.1007/978-3-030-64340-9_9

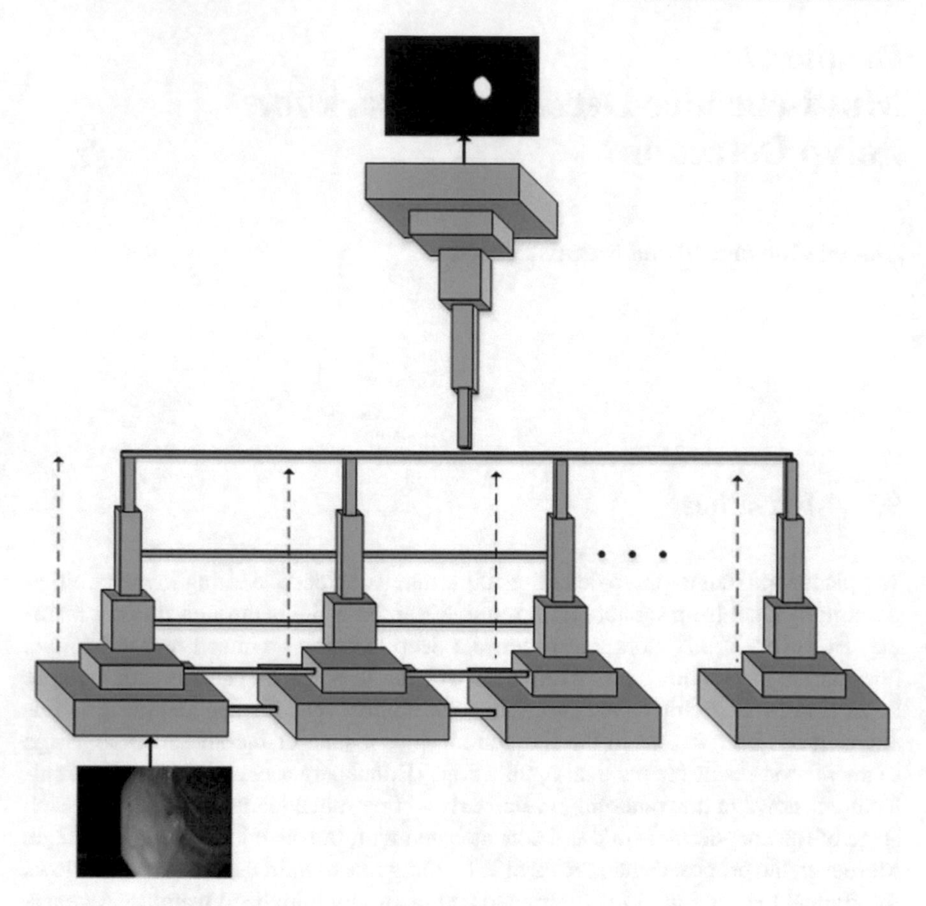

Fig. 9.1 Multi-encoder decoder object segmentation network

for having two encoders network is to address the performance loss due to domain-shift from pretrained network (natural images) to testing (polyp data), leading to degradation in performance. Since the pretrained encoder weights are initialized with VGG19 (Simonyan and Zisserman 2014), they are better suited for initializing the encoder network compared to randomly initialized weights, for extracting basic image features such as edges and curves. We propose encoder specific adaptive learning rates that update the parameters of randomly initialized encoder network with a larger step size as compared to the encoder with pretrained weights. The two encoders features are merged with a decoder network at each down-sampling path through sum-skip connection. The input to the network is an RGB video frame with the corresponding ground truth mask, and the decoder output is a binary mask segmentation of the polyp, Fig. 9.2.

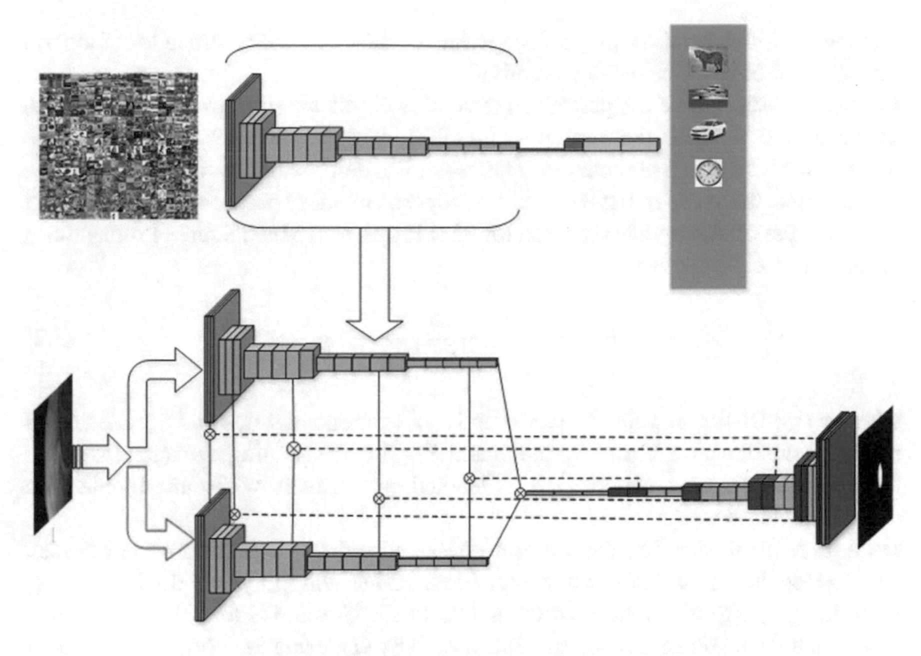

Fig. 9.2 Y-Net: given an input image, it is fed to both encoders. The weights of the last convolution at each depth of the encoder are summed and concatenated to the same spatial depth of the decoder

9.2.1 Model Learning and Implementation

Given the network architecture outlined above with one of the encoders preloaded with pretrained VGG19 weights, we explain next the optimization objectives and training strategy.

Loss function: The output layer in the decoder consists of a single plane for foreground detected polyp. We applied convolution with sigmoid activation to form the loss. Let p and g be the set of predicted and ground truth binary labels, respectively. The weighted binary cross-entropy and dice coefficient loss between two binary images is defined as

$$\mathscr{L}(p, g) = -\frac{1}{N}\sum_{i=1}^{N}\left(\frac{\lambda}{2}\cdot g_i \cdot \log p_i\right) + \left(1 - \frac{2\sum_{i=1}^{N}(g_i \cdot p_i) + \varepsilon}{\sum_{i=1}^{N}(p_i) + \sum_{i=1}^{N}(g_i) + \varepsilon}\right) \tag{9.1}$$

where λ and ε are false negatives (FN) penalty and smoothing factor, respectively In order to penalize FN more than false positives (FP) in training our network for highly imbalanced data, the first term in Eq. (9.1) penalizes FN and the second term weighs FPs and FNs (precision and recall) equally. In other words, the second term is the same as the negative of F1-score. This is to avoid miss detection of polyps, as it is more critical to miss a polyp than giving a FP. Hence, the summed loss function gives a good balance between FN and FP.

Learning rates: Since the pretrained encoder weights are initialized with VGG19, they are good, compared to randomly initialized weights, in extracting basic image features such as edges and curves. Therefore, it would be beneficial while training not to distort them too much. Hence, we propose encoder specific adaptive learning rates. The parameter update equation for RMSProp (Root Mean Square Propagation) gradient descent becomes

$$\theta_{t+1} = \theta_t - \frac{c \cdot \eta}{\sqrt{E[g^2] + \varepsilon}} \cdot g_t \tag{9.2}$$

where $c = 0.01$ for pretrained encoder and $c = 1$ for encoder two and decoder, θ is a model parameter with a learning rate η and $E[g^2]$ is the running average of squared gradients. In this way, encoder two is learned aggressively while fine-tunning the pretrained encoder.

Data augmentation: To increase robustness and reduce overfitting on our model, we increase the amount of training data. First, frames with polyp are doubled during pretraining by applying random rotation (10° to 350°), zoom (1 to 1.3), translation in x, y (–10 to 10), and shear (–25 to 25) followed by centering the polyp and cropping padded regions. Second, during training, for each frame with polyp, random cropping of the non-polyp region, as well as perspective transform, is applied with a probability of 0.3 and 0.4 with random horizontal and vertical flip, respectively. We also tried applying contrast enhancement methods such as CLAHE (Contrast-limited adaptive histogram equalization) (Zuiderveld 1994) and gamma correction, but that did not improve the detection accuracy.

Implementation Details: Our model is implemented on Tensorflow and Keras library with a single NVIDIA GeForce GTX 1080 GPU. Due to the different image sizes in the dataset, we first crop large boundary margins and resize all images into fixed dimensions with a spatial size of 224 × 224 before feeding to both encoders and finally normalized to [0, 1]. We use custom RMSProp (Eq. (9.2)) as the optimizer with batch size 3 and learning rate η set to 0.0001. We monitor the dice coefficient and use *early-stop* criteria on the validation set error.

9.3 Example of Performance

As shown in Mohammed et al. (2018), Mohammed (2019), compared to baseline architecture such as U-Net (Ronneberger et al. 2015) with VGG19 (Simon 2016) weight as encoder, Y-Net achieves a better result which suggests the multi-encoder strategy improves polyp detection accuracy. Moreover, our result suggests that hybrid fine-tuning a pretrained network and training from scratch a mirrored network gives a better performance for colonoscopy and wireless capsule endoscopy pathology detection tasks. Based on experimental results in Mohammed et al. (2018), the overall

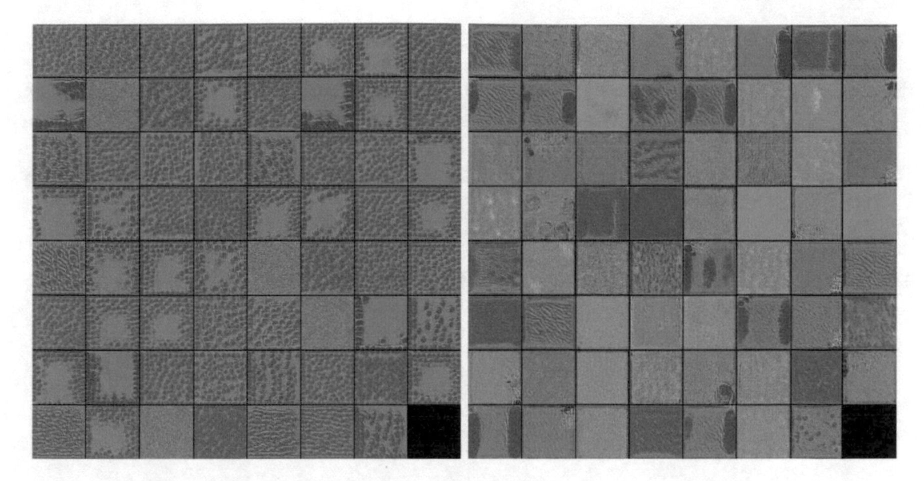

Fig. 9.3 Visualization of different layers for Y-Net. Image on the left shows the early convolutions layer in the encoder block for the first convolution. Image on the right shows late-stage convolution layer at the decoder. It is evident from patterns that the proposed model is able to learn different appearance of polyp sizes and orientation

improvement in terms of F1-score and recall is 7.3 and 13%, respectively, compared to other methods in Mohammed et al. (2018). An increase in recall metric is significant in that if a recall or true positive rate is low, it means the model misses finding polyps which can lead to a late-stage diagnosis for colorectal cancer. Elaborating on why Y-Net improves detection, we can say that it is reasonable since it uses both transfer learning and training from scratch in an end-to-end fashion it is able to improve the feature representation of the network.

Figure 9.3 shows feature responses of Y-Net at different depth of the network. The left side image shows the response of earlier layers of the encoder network. From the output, we can infer that maximum filter response is obtained for patterns having a round shape (pedunculated) with a hollow structure in the middle of the frame. The structures are similar to polyps and give a good indication that the network has learned important polyp shapes. As we move to the later stage of the model, maximum filter responses are obtained for more complicated structures with a long base similar to sessile polyps and bigger shapes.

References

Mohammed, A., Yildirim, S., Farup, I., Pedersen, M., & Hovde, Ø. (2018). Y-Net: A deep convolutional neural network for polyp detection. arXiv:1806.01907.

Mohammed, A., Yildirim, S., Farup, I., Pedersen, M., & Hovde, Ø. (2019). StreoScenNet: Surgical stereo robotic scene segmentation. *Medical Imaging 2019: Image-Guided Procedures, Robotic Interventions, and Modeling* (Vol. 10951, p. 109510P). International Society for Optics and Photonics.

Mohammed, A. K. (2019). *Computational techniques for pathology detection and quality enhancement with emphasis on colonic capsule endoscopy*. Ph.D. thesis, NTNU.

Ronneberger, O., Fischer, P., & Brox, T. (2015). U-Net: Convolutional networks for biomedical image segmentation. In *International Conference on Medical Image Computing and Computer-Assisted Intervention* (pp. 234–241). Springer.

Simon, K. (2016). Colorectal cancer development and advances in screening. *Clinical Interventions in Aging*, *11*, 967–976.

Simonyan, K., & Zisserman, A. (2014). Very deep convolutional networks for large-scale image recognition. arXiv:1409.1556.

Zuiderveld, K. (1994). Contrast limited adaptive histogram equalization. *Graphics gems* (pp. 474–485).

Chapter 10
Multi-resolution Multi-task Network and Polyp Tracking

Hanbo Chen

10.1 Motivation

Usually, different convolutional neural networks (CNN) are designed for different tasks and trained separately. However, the same convolutional encoder can be shared between classification, segmentation, and object detection network. Based on this observation, we wonder if it is possible to combine those different parts and solve multiple tasks in a single network to save the cost of training multiple networks.

Based on the observation that different tasks could rely on the same set of features, the multi-task network design could also help improve the training efficiency on small clinical dataset. Given polyp detection and localization tasks as objectives, it is likely that the attention of the CNN for positive endoscopy frame classification could also reveal the location of polyps (Liu et al. 2018; Zhou et al. 2016).

Despite multi-task constraint, supervision in middle layers has also been shown effective in improving network's performance (Merkow et al. 2016; Xie and Tu 2015). Since polyp many appear in a different size in the image (e.g., a large polyp could be small in the endoscopy image when it is far away from the camera), supervision in convolution layers with different resolutions could supervise the network in learning-related object features in different scales (Xie and Tu 2015). In addition, since the target like polyp could be sparsely distributed on the image, guidance in the low resolution feature maps can force the network giving more attention to the object of interest (Merkow et al. 2016).

Based on these previous findings, in our approach, we propose a multi-resolution multi-task network (MRMT-Net) which simultaneously conducts lesion classification, localization, and segmentation with multi-resolution guidance (Fig. 10.1). When training MRMT-Net, instead of optimizing a single objective function, a combination of multiple losses (namely, bag of losses) are simultaneously optimized. To test

H. Chen (✉)
Tencent AI Lab, 10900 NE 8th St, Bellevue, WA 98004, USA
e-mail: hanbochen@tencent.com

J. Bernal and A. Histace (eds.), *Computer-Aided Analysis of Gastrointestinal Videos*,
https://doi.org/10.1007/978-3-030-64340-9_10

MRMT-Net, we train the network to detect positive endoscopy frames, to predict the center of polyps, and to segment the area of polyps.

Notably, in this task, our goal is to detect polyp from colonoscopy videos. However, MRMT-Net and most of the other existing systems and algorithms only attempt to detect polyp in each frame separately and ignore the temporal context information in the video. By visually inspecting the result of polyp detection in each video frame with segmentation network, we noticed both false positive and false negative detection as well as jittering effect between adjacent frames. Such problem can be potentially solved by smoothing findings between adjacent frames across time.

Due to the lack of training data, it is challenging to conduct end-to-end training with temporal networks such Recurrent Neural Network. Thus, instead of introducing temporal dimension in polyp detection/segmentation network, we proposed a polyp tracking algorithm to track and smooth findings through time. In this chapter, we will first introduce MRMT-Net, which detect polyp in a single frame. Then we will introduce polyp tracking algorithm, which could process and fine-tune the results of MRMT-Net.

10.2 Introduction of the Base Structure

The design of our segmentation network is shown in Fig. 10.1. It follows U-Net architecture (Ronneberger et al. 2015). However, we heavily modified the network architecture such that we have a heavy encoder and light decoder. The idea is similar to the design of deep-lab V3 (Chen et al. 2017). For the encoder, we adopt DenseNet169 architecture (Huang et al. 2017). A three-level spatial pyramid pooling is also added on top of the DenseNet169 to hierarchically fuse global information with local information (Zhao et al. 2017). For the decoder, we repeatedly cascade a deconvolution layer (spatial resolution recover), a concatenation layer (combine feature maps of different resolutions like U-Net), and a convolution layer (fuse features in different levels). A linear interpolation layer is finally used to resize the output to the same size as input image.

Instead of using different networks for different tasks, we design the network to allow it simultaneously conduct classification, localization, and segmentation tasks (Fig. 10.1). Classification and localization results are generated based on DenseNet outputs. In addition, to facilitate detecting objects of different sizes in different scales, instead of only using the last feature map for classification, we concatenate the feature maps in the last three scales of DenseNet for the final computation.

As polyp could be of different size, to guide the network learn feature maps in different scales, we introduced multi-resolution guidance during the training. Specifically, the outputs of last three convolution layers in the encoder network are taken to train three independent classifiers. In addition to the classifiers, we also guide the training with the class activation map (CAM). The training loss of CAM is the same as segmentation loss.

10.3 Multi-resolution Guidance and Class Activation Map Supervision

In previous works, it has been shown that supervised training in the middle layers can improve the performance of segmentation networks (Merkow et al. 2016; Xie and Tu 2015) by learning features in different scales. Notably, this guidance is usually added to the layer in the decoder network. Here, we propose to add this guidance in the encoder network as a multi-resolution guidance. Specifically, the outputs of last three convolution layers in the encoder network are taken to train three independent classifiers (classifier 1–3 in Fig. 10.1). The objective function of these three classifiers is the same as the final classifier and they are computed in the same way: global average pooling layer followed by a FC layer for regression.

In addition to the classifiers, we also guide the training with the class activation map (CAM). CAM is initially proposed to visualize the activated image regions associated with classification decisions (Zhou et al. 2016). Given a CNN ended with global average pooling and a FC layer, by taking the parameters w in the FC layer as the weight factor of the output channels h_i in the last convolution layer of CNN, the CAM of an image is defined as

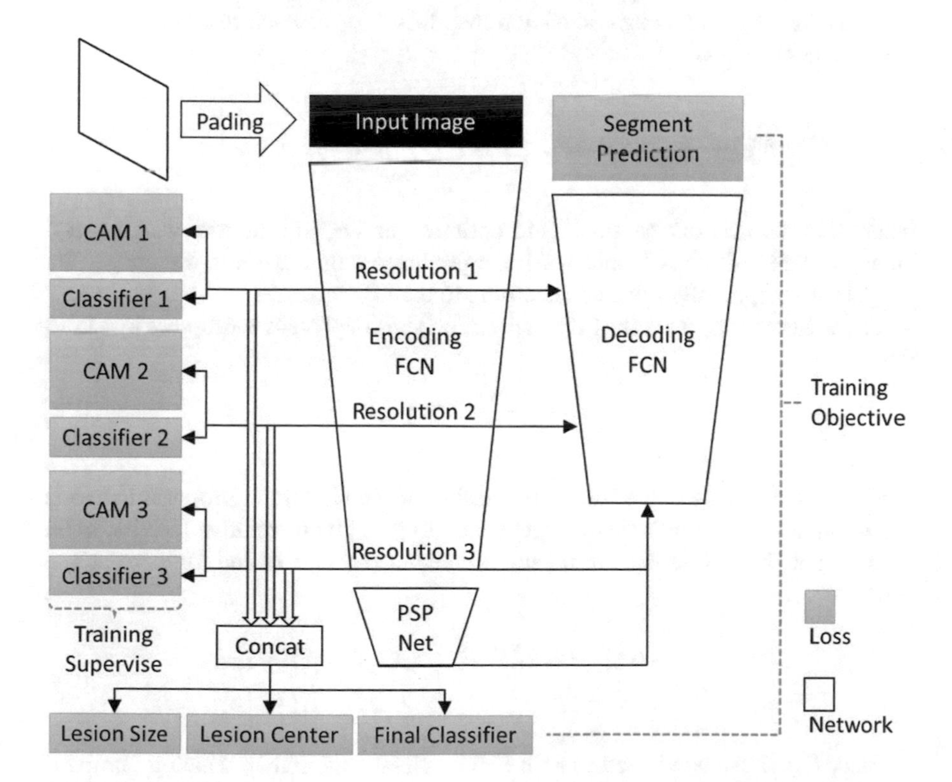

Fig. 10.1 Detailed architecture of multi-resolution multi-task supervised segmentation network

$$CAM(x, \theta) = b + a \sum_{i=0}^{N} w_i h_i \tag{10.1}$$

where h_i and w_i are the hidden variables of channel i and the corresponding FC layer weight. a and b are the shift and scaling factors to normalize CAM.

Usually, when CAM agrees with the semantic segmentation of the class, it indicates that the classifier correctly learns the features associated with that class. Later, it has been shown that by taking CAM as optimization objective like segmentation tasks can also improve the performance of a classifier (Li et al. 2018). Inspired by this observation, we further optimize CAM of multi-resolution classifiers in our training process. The shifting and scaling factors (a and b) in Eq. 10.1 are optimized together.

10.4 Bag of Losses

As highlighted by gray-boxes in Fig. 10.1, MRMT-Net has nine optimization objectives. In summary, they are loss of final classifier L_c, loss of target center regressor L_l, loss of segmentation L_s, and the multi-resolution guidance loss L_{MR} including classifier loss $L_{(i,c)}$ and class activation map loss $L_{(i,a)}$ in each resolution. We call them a bag of losses:

$$(\theta) = \arg\min_{\theta} \alpha_c L_c + \mu \alpha_l L_l + \alpha_s L_s + \sum_{i=1}^{3} (\alpha_{i,c} L_{i,c} + \alpha_{i,a} L_{i,a}) \tag{10.2}$$

where θ is the network parameters to optimize, and α_* are the loss weights. μ is binary variable which is 1 only when the predicted target exists in the image. The weights are empirically selected according to their importance.

For all classifiers, we follow the convention and adapt cross-entropy as loss function:

$$L_c = -\sum_{k}^{C} \log(y_{c,k}) \tag{10.3}$$

For center regressor, we follow the design of classic region proposal networks and normalize the coordinate of target center to [0, 1] by its relative location in the image. Then the smooth-L1 norm between predicted center y_l^* and truth center y_l is computed:

$$L_l = \begin{cases} 0.5||y_l^* - y_l||^2 & \text{if } |y_l^* - y_l| \leq 1, \\ |y_l^* - y_l| & \text{if } |y_l^* - y_l| > 1, \end{cases} \tag{10.4}$$

Since CAM can be viewed as a pixel-wise classification map which is similar to segmentation map, the same loss function is utilized to compute the dissimilarity between predicted segmentation/CAM y_s^* and the truth segmentation y_s. To deal with the sparsely distributed foreground object in our problem, we combine dice coefficient with cross-entropy when computing the segmentation loss:

$$L_s = -\gamma \sum [y_s \log(y_s^*) + (1 - y_s) \log(1 - y_s^*)] - \mu(2 \sum y_s \cdot y_s^*)/(\sum (y_s + y_s^*)) \tag{10.5}$$

where γ is the trade-off value, and μ is the binary variable in Eq. 10.2 which zeros-out dice loss when the mask is empty.

10.5 Polyp Tracking Algorithm

In our solution, we first identify polyp detection with high confidence and only keep them at the beginning. Then we adopted a tracking algorithm to track the detected polyp and smooth the polyp detection through time (Zheng et al. 2019) (Fig. 10.2). The rationale behind this design is based on the following three observations: (1) the location of polyp is consistent between adjacent frames; (2) the appearance of one polyp is consistent in the videos; (3) only 1 polyp can be observed in a frame in most of the times. The system is composed by three critical steps and will be elaborated in details: (1) confident polyp seed detection; (2) object tracking; and (3) spatial voting.

To find the polyp detection with high confidence, we averaged segmentation map by different weights through the time:

$$S_i = \sum_{j=1}^{N} \gamma^{|i-j|} V_j M_j \tag{10.6}$$

where S_i is the averaged segmentation map of frame i, M_j is the raw segmentation map of frame j, V_j is the likelihood ratio of frame j be classified as positive frame, γ is the decaying factor of time which we set to 0.5 in this work.

The pixels with high value in S_i meet the following three criteria and thus can be taken with high confidence as polyp detected: (1) The frame has high likelihood to be positive, (2) the pixel has high likelihood to be segmented as foreground, (3) both criteria are consistent over the time. We then threshold S_i with a relatively high value and took the center of the largest connected component inside a frame as a confident polyp seed.

We track the polyp seed across frames to complete the missing ones. Given a polyp p_i^j in frame j, the goal is to compute p_i^{j+1}. Optical tracking is adopt to fulfill the task (Lucas and Kanade 1981). However, it may fail and lost the target when motion is large. As a back up, we adopt on-the-fly trained CNN to track the polyp (Chu et al. 2017). In brief, four image crops close to p_i^j are taken as positive samples and other four crops far away are taken as negative samples. An CNN is trained to classify them. The CNN then classify crops on frame $j+1$ to search for p_i^{j+1}. If none of the crops meet the criteria, the tracking of p_i will be terminated.

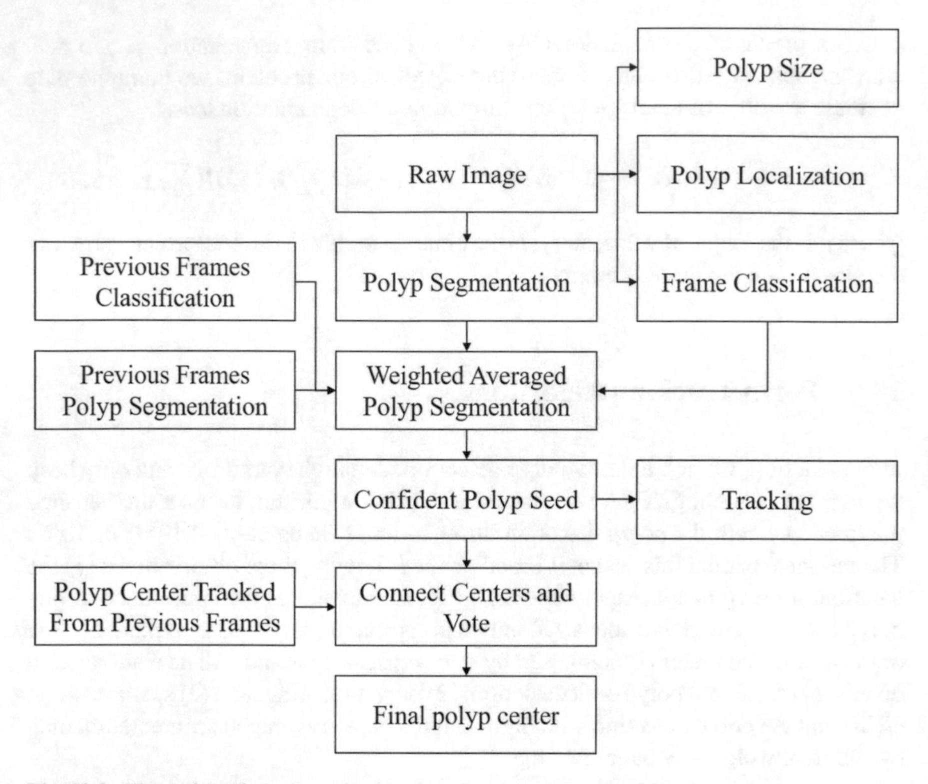

Fig. 10.2 Illustration of pipeline of polyp detection in endoscopic video stream

For the same polyp, seeds could be generated on multiple frames. After tracking, there could be multiple tracked polyp center on the same frame. Based on the assumption that only one polyp should be observed each time, we filter outliers and combine the rest into the final one. In practice, the centers with distance smaller than threshold are connected. Then the center of the largest component is taken as the final result.

10.6 Data Normalization and Augmentation

Given that the number of training data is limited, to avoid over-fit, we first normalized the data into a uniform space and then augment the data during training (Fig. 10.3). During the testing phase, only normalization will take place.

Normalization is performed in the following order: (1) crop the blanket border in the image; (2) isotropically resize image and zero-pad the shorter edge to uniform size; (3) shift the average hue and the saturation of image to the same value.

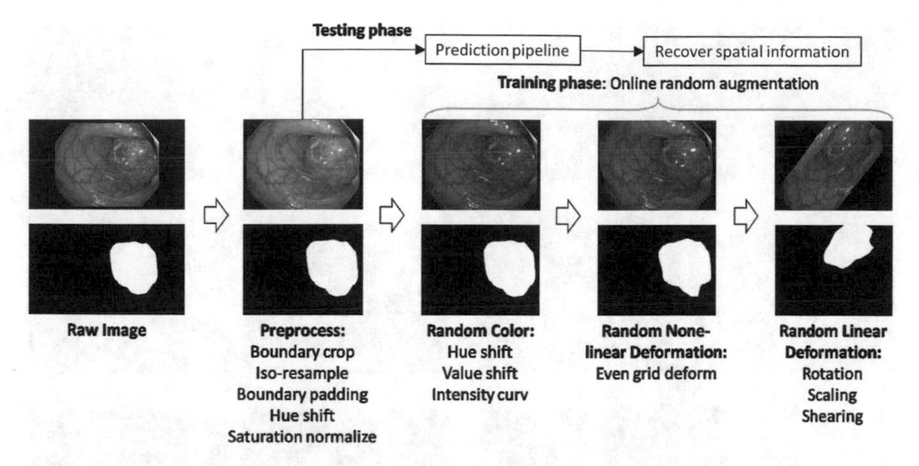

Fig. 10.3 Illustration of data pre-processing and training augmentation pipeline

Augmentation is performed in the following order with parameters given in the bracelet: (1) random hue shift (±20); (2) random value shift (±20); (3) random intensity scale by curve; (4) random deformation; (5) random rotation (180°); (6) random scaling (±20%); (7) random shearing (±20°).

10.7 Example of Results

In Fig. 10.4, we visualize some example results of MRMT-Net predictions. By visual inspection, the predicted result largely agrees with annotation truth. Moreover, as highlighted by the white arrows in Fig. 10.4e, f, our model also detects potential polyps that were missed by human experts when annotating. And for these two cases that contain two polyps, the polyp center regressor still correctly localizes the position of the primary findings.

In comparison with single frame detection system, the proposed tracking system can significant improve recall value. However, since increasing the number of polyp detected also increases the chance of false positive detection, we observed a small trade-in of precision value. The balance between false positive and false negative findings can be fine-tuned by changing the confidence threshold to control the number of tracking seeds. In our result, the overall F1 and F2 scores are higher than single frame detector. For more details, one can refer to Zheng et al. (2019).

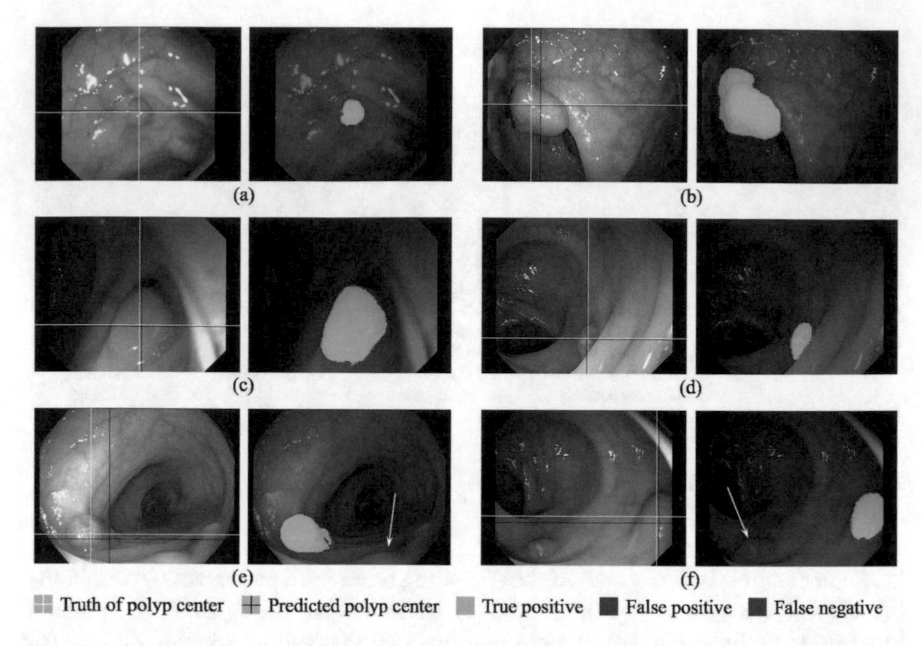

Fig. 10.4 Six examples of prediction results by our proposed method. On the left side of each sub-figure shows the raw image overlapped with polyp center truth (white cross) and predicted polyp center (black cross). On the right side of each sub-figure is the comparison between predicted segmentation and the truth annotation overlaid on the dimmed raw image. White arrows pointing to potential polyps missed by human experts when annotating

References

Chen, L.-C., Papandreou, G., Schroff, F., & Adam, H. (2017). Rethinking atrous convolution for semantic image segmentation. arXiv:1706.05587.

Chu, Q., Ouyang, W., Li, H., Wang, X., Liu, B., & Yu, N. (2017). Online multi-object tracking using CNN-based single object tracker with spatial-temporal attention mechanism. In *Proceedings of the IEEE International Conference on Computer Vision* (pp. 4836–4845).

Huang, G., Liu, Z., Van Der Maaten, L., & Weinberger, K. Q. (2017). Densely connected convolutional networks. In *Proceedings of the IEEE Conference on Computer Vision and Pattern Recognition* (pp. 4700–4708).

Li, K., Wu, Z., Peng, K.-C., Ernst, J., & Fu, Y. (2018). Tell me where to look: Guided attention inference network. In *Proceedings of the IEEE Conference on Computer Vision and Pattern Recognition* (pp. 9215–9223).

Liu, J., Li, W., Zhao, N., Cao, K., Yin, Y., Song, Q., et al. (2018). Integrate domain knowledge in training CNN for ultrasonography breast cancer diagnosis. In *International Conference on Medical Image Computing and Computer-Assisted Intervention* (pp. 868–875). Springer.

Lucas, B. D., & Kanade, T. (1981). An iterative image registration technique with an application to stereo vision. In *Proceedings DARPA Image Understanding* (p. 121430).

Merkow, J., Marsden, A., Kriegman, D., & Tu, Z. (2016). Dense volume-to-volume vascular boundary detection. In *International Conference on Medical Image Computing and Computer-Assisted Intervention* (pp. 371–379). Springer.

Ronneberger, O., Fischer, P., & Brox, T. (2015). U-Net: Convolutional networks for biomedical image segmentation. In *International Conference on Medical Image Computing and Computer-Assisted Intervention* (pp. 234–241). Springer.

Xie, S., & Tu, Z. (2015). Holistically-nested edge detection. In *Proceedings of the IEEE International Conference on Computer Vision* (pp. 1395–1403).

Zhao, H., Shi, J., Qi, X., Wang, X., & Jia, J. (2017). Pyramid scene parsing network. In *Proceedings of the IEEE Conference on Computer Vision and Pattern Recognition* (pp. 2881–2890).

Zheng, H., Chen, H., Huang, J., Li, X., Han, X., & Yao, J. (2019). Polyp tracking in video colonoscopy using optical flow with an on-the-fly trained CNN. In *2019 IEEE 16th International Symposium on Biomedical Imaging (ISBI 2019)* (pp. 79–82). IEEE.

Zhou, B., Khosla, A., Lapedriza, A., Oliva, A., & Torralba, A. (2016). Learning deep features for discriminative localization. In *Proceedings of the IEEE Conference on Computer Vision and Pattern Recognition* (pp. 2921–2929).

Chapter 11
Region-Based Convolutional Neural Network for Polyp Detection and Segmentation

Hemin Ali Qadir, Ilangko Balasingham, and Younghak Shin

11.1 Introduction

For polyp detection, we adapt a Faster R-CNN (Ren et al. 2015) architecture shown in Fig. 11.1. Faster R-CNN has two stages: region proposal network (RPN), and a box classifier network. Both stages share a common set of convolutional layers as a feature extractor to reduce the marginal cost for detection. The RPN utilizes feature maps of the last convolutional layer to generate class-agnostic RoI proposals called *anchors*, each with an objectness confidence value. The anchors have different aspect ratios and scales. The classifier network crops these anchors from the feature maps of the last convolutional layer and feeds the cropped features to the remainder of the network in order to predict location and confidence values of the object class (polyps). We use Inception-ResNet-v2 (Szegedy et al. 2017) as the feature extractor which was pre-trained on Microsoft's COCO dataset (Lin et al. 2014). For polyp segmentation, we use Mask R-CNN (He et al. 2017) which is a general framework for object instance segmentation. Mask R-CNN is an intuitive extension of Faster R-CNN (see Fig. 11.1). It has the same structure of Faster R-CNN with an extra branch to the second stage for predicting polyp masks in parallel with the existing branches

H. A. Qadir · I. Balasingham
The Intervention Centre, Oslo University Hospital, Sognsvannsveien 20, 0372 Oslo, Norway
e-mail: hemina.qadir@gmail.com

I. Balasingham
e-mail: ilangko.balasingham@ntnu.no

I. Balasingham
Department of Electronic Systems, NTNU, Norwegian University of Science and Technology, Høgskoleringen 1, 7491 Trondheim, Norway

Y. Shin (✉)
Department of Computer Engineering, Mokpo National University, 1666, Yeongsan-ro, Cheonggye-myeon, Jeollanam-do, Republic of Korea
e-mail: shinyh0919@gmail.com

J. Bernal and A. Histace (eds.), *Computer-Aided Analysis of Gastrointestinal Videos*,
https://doi.org/10.1007/978-3-030-64340-9_11

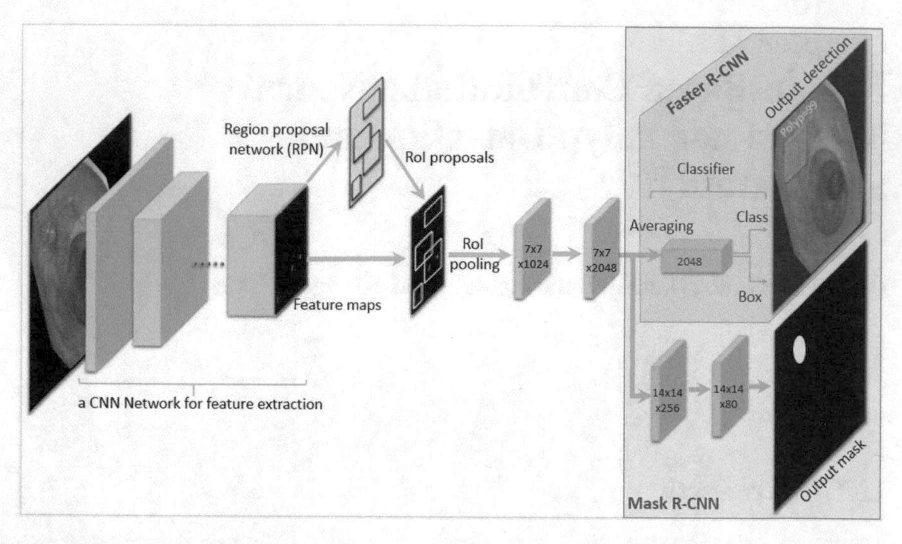

Fig. 11.1 Faster R-CNN and Mask R-CNN architecture used for polyp detection and segmentation, respectively. They both share the same structure except there is an additional branch to predict mask in Mask R-CNN as highlighted in light blue

for bounding box regression and confidence value. Instead of using RoIPool, which performs coarse quantization for feature extraction in Faster R-CNN, Mask R-CNN uses RoIAlign, quantization-free layer, to fix the misalignment problem. For further improvement, we combine outputs of two Mask R-CNNs with two different feature extractor networks, i.e., Inception-ResNet-v2 (Szegedy et al. 2017) and ResNet 101 (He et al. 2016) both pre-trained on Microsoft's COCO dataset (Lin et al. 2014).

11.2 ResNet 101 and Inception-ResNet-v2

ResNet stands for residual networks. It is proposed by Kaiming He et al. (2016) to address the degradation problem associated with deeper networks. Deeper networks are crucial for performance improvement. Higher levels of features can be extracted by adding more stacked layers. However, training a deeper network with more layers becomes problematic due to vanishing or exploding gradients problem. In ResNet, there are skip connections to prevent gradients from vanishing/exploding during training. The skip connection enables to have deeper networks and benefit from rich features, and thus better performance can be achieved. Figure 11.2 shows how skip connection is formed and solves the problem of vanishing and exploding gradients.

Hence, the output is a combination of x and $f(x)$

$$h(x) = f(x) + x, \tag{11.1}$$

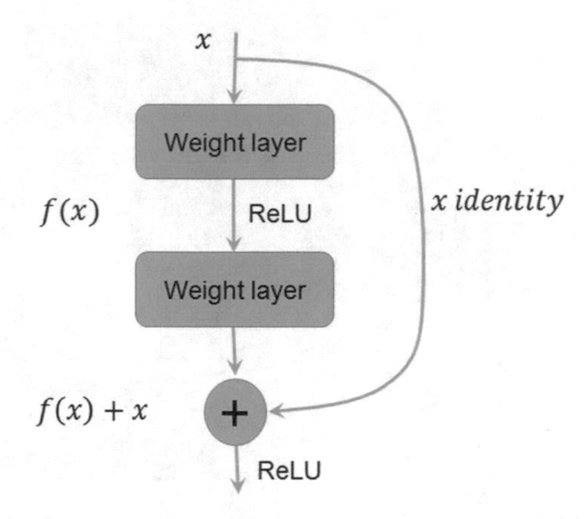

Fig. 11.2 A building block of residual network

the weight layers learns a kind of residual mapping

$$f(x) = h(x) - x, \tag{11.2}$$

that means there is always the identity (x) to transfer back to earlier layers, even if there is vanishing gradients.

ResNet 101 has 101 layers in the form of residual connections shown in Fig. 11.2. Its full architecture can be found in Table 1 in He et al. (2016). ResNet 101 achieved 4.60% top-5 error on the ImageNet validation dataset for classification. We use ResNet 101 as the feature extractor network for our Mask R-CNN of auxiliary model (see Sect. 11.4).

Inception architecture was proposed by C. Szegedy et al. in Szegedy et al. (2015) to allow for increasing the depth and width of the network for better performance at relatively low computational cost. Inception module tries to create a sparse structure using dense components of convolutional layers as shown in Fig. 11.3. C. Szegedy et al. in Szegedy et al. (2017) showed that training of Inception networks can significantly be accelerated with residual connections. They also presented that residual Inception networks could outperform counterpart Inception networks without residual. We use Inception-ResNet-v2 (see Fig. 15 in Szegedy et al. (2017)) as our feature extractor network for Faster R-CNN and Mask R-CNN of our main model. This network combines the benefits from both Inception-v4 architecture (see Fig. 9 in Szegedy et al. (2017)) and residual connections in a single network. We choose this network because it outperformed its variants (Inception-v3, Inception-ResNet-v1 and Inception-v4) on ImageNet validation dataset.

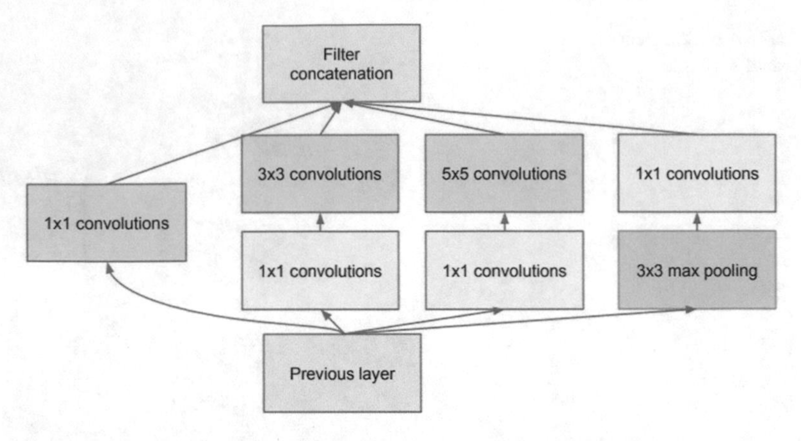

Fig. 11.3 Inception module (Szegedy et al. 2015)

11.3 Polyp Detection

Current deep neural networks, including CNNs, are vulnerable to small noises and can easily be fooled (Su et al. 2019). In colonoscopy, Faster R-CNN might get fooled by the specular highlights and small changes in polyp appearance. This means that the same polyp appearing in a sequence of neighboring frames might be missed and unstable detection output contaminated with a high number of FPs will be produced by Faster R-CNN. We use temporal dependencies among consecutive frames to find and remove FPs and detect intra-frame missed polyps based on the consecutive detection outputs of Faster R-CNN. Neighboring frames should contain the same polyp with slight changes in its position and size.

Our method for polyp detection consists of two stages as illustrated in Fig. 11.4: (1) the Faster R-CNN shown in Fig. 11.1 to provide region of interests (RoI), (2) a false positive (FP) reduction unit to explore the temporal dependencies among neighboring frames. The Faster R-CNN proposes multiple RoIs to the FP reduction unit. The FP reduction unit exploits the temporal dependencies among the neighboring frames in video by integrating the bidirectional temporal information obtained by RoIs in a set of consecutive frames. This information is used to make the final decision.

We let Faster R-CNN to provide one RoI per frame. We set the confidence threshold value of Faster R-CNN to 0.0 so that we always have a RoI regardless of its confidence value in every frame. The proposed RoIs in a number of previous and future frames are passed through the FP reduction unit to find detection irregularities and outliers before the final decision is made for the RoI in the current frame—the frame in the middle. When a polyp appears in a sequence of frames, its location slightly changes following a motion estimating the movement in the sequence. Irregularities and outliers are those detection outputs that do not smoothly follow such a movement. We consider those detection irregularities and outliers as FPs. In case of an outlier, we use interpolation (Lagrange formula) to correct the detection. There-

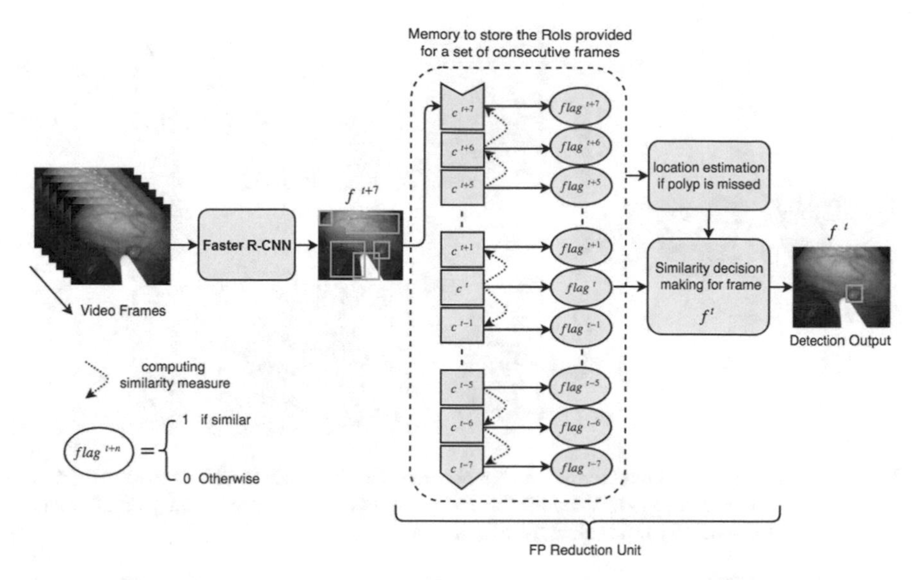

Fig. 11.4 Our proposed method for polyp detection. The Faster R-CNN provides RoIs to the FP reduction unit. The FP reduction unit classifies the RoIs as either TPs or FPs using temporal coherence information among a set of consecutive frames, and estimates the location of missed polyps using interpolation

fore, the FP reduction unit comprises of two processes: a mechanism to detect FPs, and a mechanism to correct the outliers denoting the missed polyps in the sequence.

We only pick those RoIs overlapped with at least 7 RoIs in a set of 15 consecutive frames, i.e., 7 previous frames and 7 future frames (optimized numbers). We also calculate the average confidence for the overlapped RoIs and only classify those RoIs with an average confidence $(avg - th) \geq 0.5$ as TPs. In this way, we have less FPs and keep only those RoIs that repeat in more than 7 consecutive frames with high confidence values in the final output.

11.4 Polyp Segmentation

Dissimilar CNN feature extractors compute different types of features due to differences in their number of layers and architectures. A deeper CNN can extract higher levels of features from the input images while it loses some spatial information due to the contraction and pooling layers. To segment polyps from normal mucosa, we propose an ensemble Mask R-CNN shown in Fig. 11.5. We combine results of two Mask R-CNN models with two different CNN feature extractors, i.e., Inception-ResNet-v2 and ResNet 101. The hypothesis is that some polyps might be missed by one of the models while they could be detected by the other one. We use Mask R-CNN with Inception-ResNet-v2 as the main model and its output is always relied on. We use

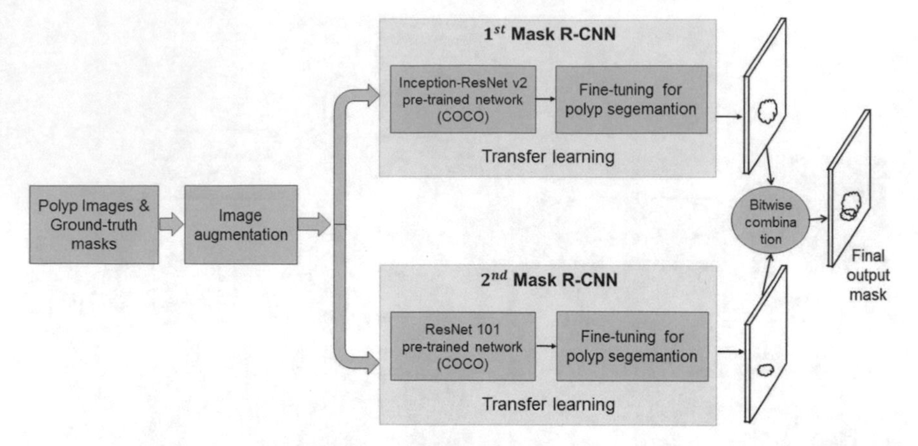

Fig. 11.5 Our proposed method for polyp segmentation. The first Mask R-CNN is used as the main model and its output is always taken while the second Mask R-CNN is used as an auxiliary model to help detect missed polyps and refine the output masks

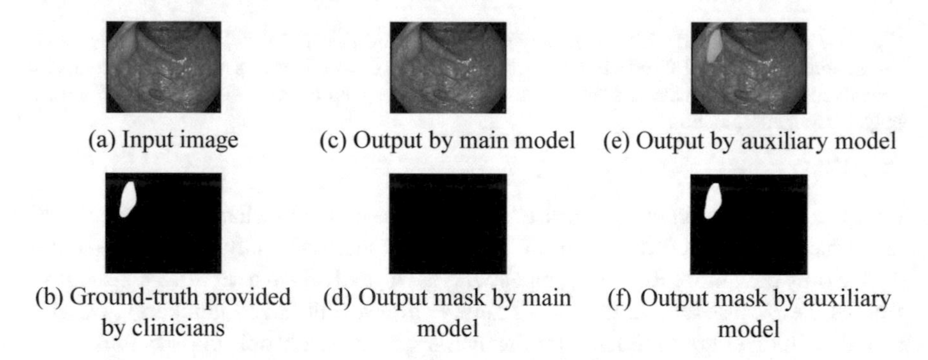

Fig. 11.6 A case which explains the benefit of our ensemble model

Mask R-CNN with ResNet 101 as an auxiliary model to support the main model. To avoid increasing FPs, we only take into account the outputs from the auxiliary model when the confidence of the detection is >95% (an optimized value using a validation dataset).

Figure 11.6 illustrates a case where a polyp in the input image is missed by Mask R-CNN with Inception-ResNet-v2 while it is successfully detected and segmented by Mask R-CNN with ResNet 101. It is also possible that a polyp might be partially segmented by the main model and precisely segmented by the auxiliary model to complete the final segmentation and vise versa.

Table 11.1 Augmentation strategies applied to enlarge the training dataset

Augmentation	Quantity	Applied to
Rotation	90, 180 and 270 degrees	Original images
Flip	Horizontal and vertical	Original images
Shearing	Two alone x-axis and two alone y-axis	Original images
Zoom-in	10% only	Riginal+rotated+flipped
Zoom-out	(10, 30, and 50)%	Original+rotated+flipped

11.5 Training the Systems

11.5.1 Augmentations and Fine-Tuning

It is important to mention that we only use those images (frames) that contain at least one polyp. ResNet 101 and Inception-ResNet-v2 are deep and complex networks. The datasets of polyps provided for GIANA challenge are not large enough to train such deep networks. Therefore, we apply augmentation strategies to enlarge the training data and prevent the models from overfitting. This augmentation step cannot improve data distribution, i.e., it can only add an image-level transformation through depth and scale. Table 11.1 presents all the augmentation techniques that we apply to increase training data for both Faster R-CNN and Mask R-CNN.

Only applying augmentation does not ensure the models from being overfitted. Therefore, we use transfer learning by initializing the weights of Resnet 101 and Inception-ResNet-v2 from models pre-trained on Microsoft's COCO for both tasks.

We use stochastic gradient descent (SGD) with a momentum of 0.9, learning rate of 0.0003, and batch size of 1 to fine-tune the pre-trained models using the augmented datasets. We keep the original image size during both training and test phases.

11.5.2 Objective Losses

To train our Faster R-CNN, we use a combined loss of classification loss ℓ_{cls} for the predicted class $f_{cls}(I; a, \theta)$ (polyp or background) and location loss ℓ_{loc} for the predicted bounding box $f_{loc}(I; a, \theta)$ on each *anchor* proposed by RPN. If intersection of union (IoU) between anchor a and ground-truth box b is > 0.3, then anchor a is considered as a positive anchor, and we assign a class label $y_a = 1$, and a vector $(\phi(b_a; a))$ encoding box b with respect to anchor a. If IoU is < 0.3, anchor a is considered as a negative sample, and the class label is set to $y_a = 0$,

$$\mathcal{L}(a, I; \theta) = \frac{1}{m}\sum_{i=1}^{m}\frac{1}{N}\sum_{j=1}^{N}\alpha \cdot 1[a \textit{ is positive}] \cdot \ell_{loc}\left(\phi(b_a; a) - f_{loc}(I; a, \theta)\right) + \beta \cdot \ell_{cls}\left(y_a, f_{cls}(I; a, \theta)\right). \tag{11.3}$$

For Mask R-CNN, we add the mask branch which has a 14×14-dimensional output for each anchor. Then the loss for each anchor a consists of three losses: location loss ℓ_{loc}, classification loss ℓ_{cls}, and mask loss ℓ_{mask} for the predicted mask $f_{mask}(I, a, \theta)$,

$$\mathcal{L}(a, I; \theta) = \frac{1}{m}\sum_{i=1}^{m}\frac{1}{N}\sum_{j=1}^{N} 1[a \textit{ is positive}] \cdot \ell_{loc}\left(\phi(b_a; a) - f_{loc}(I; a, \theta)\right) + \ell_{cls}\left(y_a, f_{cls}(I; a, \theta)\right) + \ell_{mask}\left(mask_a, f_{mask}(I, a, \theta)\right). \tag{11.4}$$

In both Eqs. (11.3) and (11.4), I is the image, θ is the model parameters, m is the size of mini-batch and N is the number of anchors for each frame. We use softmax for the classification loss, Smooth L1 for the localization loss, and binary cross-entropy for the mask loss.

References

He, K., Gkioxari, G., Dollár, P., & Girshick, R. (2017). Mask r-cnn.

He, K., Zhang, X., Ren, S., & Sun, J. (2016). Deep residual learning for image recognition. In *Proceedings of the IEEE Conference on Computer Vision and Pattern Recognition* (pp. 770–778).

Lin, T.-Y., Maire, M., Belongie, S., Hays, J., Perona, P., Ramanan, D., Dollár, P., & Zitnick, C. L. (2014). Microsoft coco: Common objects in context. In *European Conference on Computer Vision* (pp. 740–755). Springer.

Ren, S., He, K., Girshick, R., & Sun, J. (2015). Faster r-cnn: Towards real-time object detection with region proposal networks. In *Advances in neural information processing systems* (pp. 91–99).

Su, J., Vargas, D. V., & Sakurai, K. (2019). One pixel attack for fooling deep neural networks. *IEEE Transactions on Evolutionary Computation*.

Szegedy, C., Ioffe, S., Vanhoucke, V., & Alemi, A. A. (2017). Inception-v4, inception-resnet and the impact of residual connections on learning. In *Thirty-First AAAI Conference on Artificial Intelligence*.

Szegedy, C., Liu, W., Jia, Y., Sermanet, P., Reed, S., Anguelov, D., Erhan, D., Vanhoucke, V., & Rabinovich, A. (2015). Going deeper with convolutions. In *Proceedings of the IEEE Conference on Computer Vision and Pattern Recognition* (pp. 1–9).

Chapter 12
ResNet

Isabel Amaya-Rodriguez, Isabel Amaya-Rodriguez, Javier Civit-Masot, Francisco Luna-Perejon, Lourdes Duran-Lopez, Alexander Rakhlin, Sergey Nikolenko, Satoshi Kondo, Pablo Laiz, Jordi Vitrià, Santi Seguí, and Patrick Brandao

12.1 General Motivation

In this chapter, all groups have used Residual Network (ResNet) (He et al. 2016) as part of different architectures with the purpose of solving the GIANA challenge. In some cases like RTC-ATC group ResNet-50 was used as a layer in Faster Convolutional Neural Network (FCNN) in order to build an automated recognition system to detect the presence of polyps in colonoscopy images.

The main reason to use this network is because ResNet models try to solve the overload of the accuracy which comes from network depth. The accuracy saturation is not due to overfitting or the quantity of layers is because of the named Vanishing Gradient (Hochreiter 1998) this effect try to explain when the network is deep the loss functions in gradients value are near to zero after several chain rule applications. Then weights are not updated and consequently no learning is being performed. To

I. Amaya-Rodriguez (✉)
Vicomtech, Paseo Mikeletegi 57, Donostia-San Sebastian, Spain
e-mail: iamaya@vicomtech.com

I. Amaya-Rodriguez · J. Civit-Masot · F. Luna-Perejon · L. Duran-Lopez
Robotics and Computer Technology Lab., University of Seville, Seville, Spain

A. Rakhlin · S. Nikolenko
Steklov Institute of Mathematics at St. Petersburg, Russia nab. r. Fontanki, 27, St. Petersburg 191023, Russia

S. Kondo
Konica Minolta, Inc., 1-2 Sakura-machi, Takatsuki, Osaka 569-8503, Japan

P. Laiz · J. Vitrià · S. Seguí
Departament de Matemàtiques i Informàtica de la Universitat de Barcelona, Barcelona, Spain

P. Brandao
Wellcome/EPSRC Centre for Interventional & Surgical Sciences, University College London, London, UK

J. Bernal and A. Histace (eds.), *Computer-Aided Analysis of Gastrointestinal Videos*,
https://doi.org/10.1007/978-3-030-64340-9_12

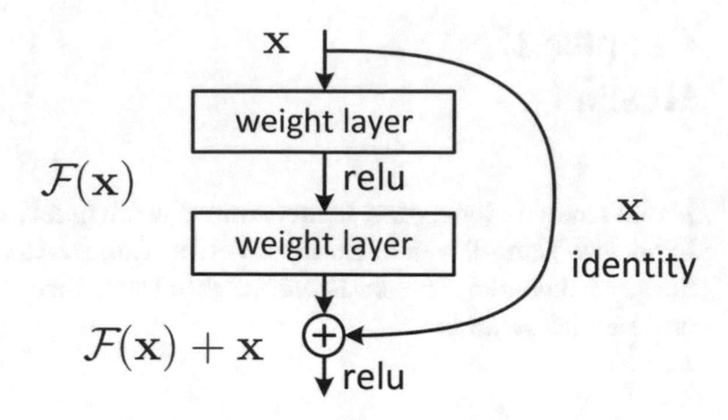

Fig. 12.1 Residual learning block

solve this problem, Microsoft created a new deep learning concept based on residual leaning which allows gradients to flow between layers.

12.2 Introduction to ResNet Architecture

In this section, the basic concepts of ResNet architecture is explained. As it was introduced in the Sect. 12.1 ResNet architecture makes it possible to implement hundreds or even thousands of layers and still achieves compelling performance. Residual Network works substracting features learned from input of that layer.

The main characteristic introduced by ResNet is the identity shortcut connection defined as $F(x) := H(x) - x$ shown in Fig. 12.1. This shortcut connections X are identity mappings and their outputs are added to the following stacked layers. Then ResNet apply simply stacked identity mappings and the residual of X in H(x) is learned. It solves problems like training error increase when the depth increases too.

In the case of ResNet-12 contains five Residual Blocks as shows Fig. 12.2. For each two-convolutional layer there is one identity shorcut connection.

12.3 Methodologies

12.3.1 RTC-ATC Group

In this section, RTC-ATC group shows an application of Faster R-CNNs (FRCNN) in order to build an automated recognition system to detect the presence of polyps in colonoscopy images presented in GIANA challenge 2019. To realize this goal, they used an implementation of FRCNN with ResNet-50 as Fully Convolutional Network (FCN) architecture. FRCNN builds on the idea of Region Proposals by sharing intermediate features with the classification network. For example, the ResNet takes an

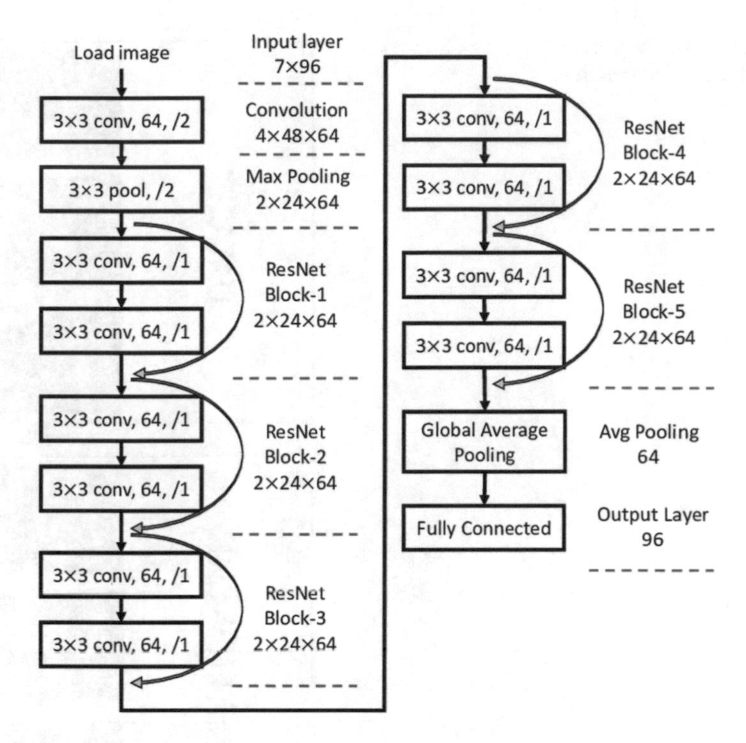

Fig. 12.2 ResNet-12 architecture

input image and produces a series of transformations before arriving at the prediction. The FRCNN will use the intermediate features of ResNet to aid in region proposal.

12.3.1.1 Brief Methodology Introduction

Faster R-CNNs have been used for different purposes: face detection (Jiang and Learned-Miller 2017), driver's cell-phone usage and hands on steering wheel detection (Hoang Ngan Le et al. 2016) are some application examples of this algorithm, which has proven to show good results. As it was mentioned in the introduction, a FRCNN was used in this work for the polyp detection task. This algorithm is divided into two modules (Fig. 12.3):

1. First of all, a deep Fully Convolutional Network (FCN) (Ren et al. 2015) receives the images from the dataset. Then, it extracts feature maps or descriptive characteristics and analyzes them to propose regions of interest. The novel step that this architecture introduced is the way to determine the regions of interest. Region Proposal Network (RPN) is computed base on the output feature map of the previous step. Then, RPN is connected to a convolutional layer with 3×3 filters, 1 padding, 512 output channels. The output is connected to two 1×1 convo-

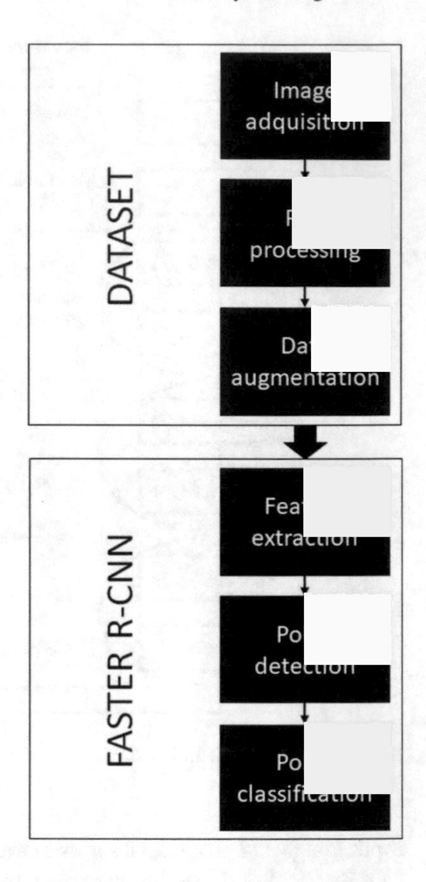

Fig. 12.3 Block diagram of the implemented approach

lutional layer for classification and box-regression (Note that the classification here is to determine if the box is an object or not).

2. Next, as shows Fig. 12.4 ROI pooling layer is used for these proposed regions in order to ensure the standard and pre-defined output size. These valid outputs are passed to a fully connected layer as inputs. In our case, by using a neural network that takes advantage of the mathematical operations made in the convolutional layers. In our architecture we have used the ResNet-50 model (He et al. 2016) as FCN. ResNet models try to solve the saturation of the accuracy caused by increasing the network depth (Fig. 12.5).
3. Finally, the proposed regions that are the input of the second module, called Fast R-CNN detector, composed of two fully connected layers, a regression layer and a classification layer (Ren et al. 2015).

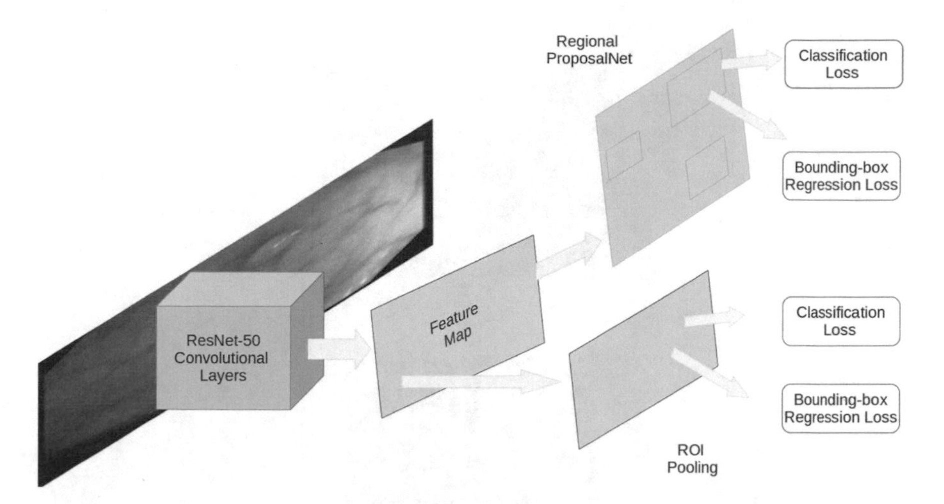

Fig. 12.4 ResNet-50 in faster convolutional neural network

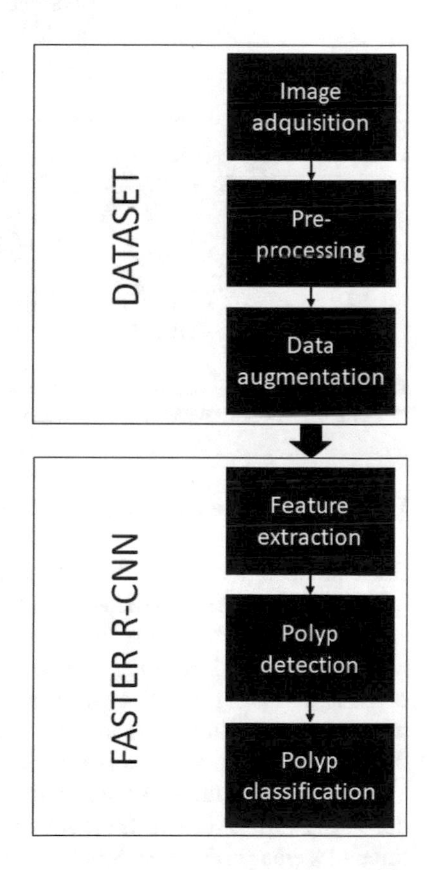

Fig. 12.5 Block diagram of the implemented approach

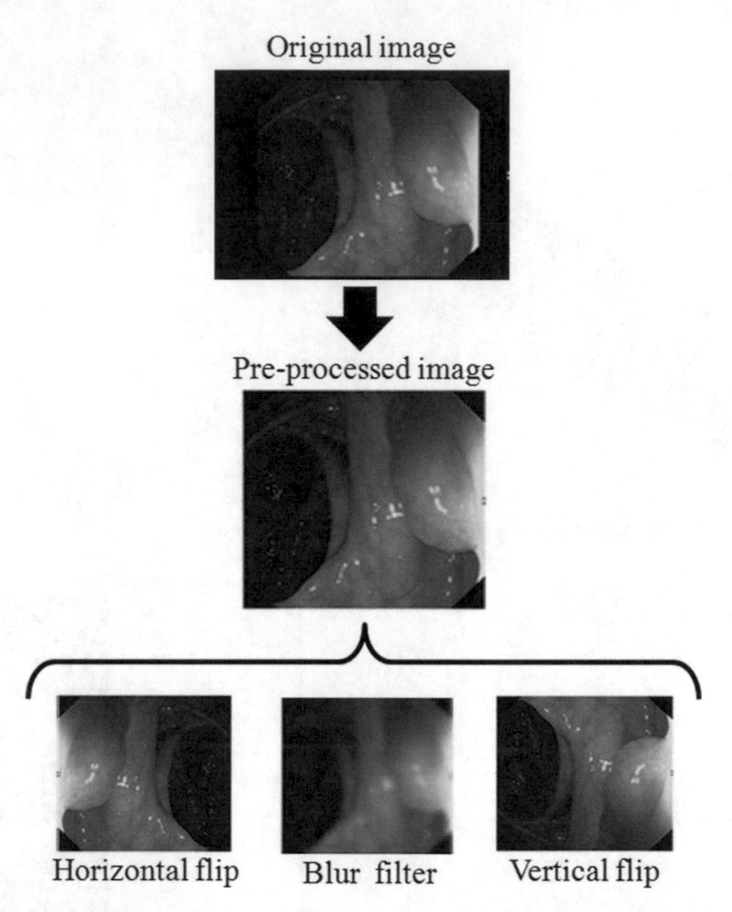

Fig. 12.6 Processing applied to the original images. First, black edges are removed in a pre-processing step. Then data augmentation is applied, generating three different new images

12.3.1.2 Architecture and Parameters Tuning

Basic architecture was modified to achieve the better results, aiming to observe the benefit of using different datasets by training the network with background examples and augmented dataset. Firstly, with the aim of reducing the number of false positives, a technique called hard-negative mining was used (Felzenszwalb et al. 2009). It consists of adding negative samples, which means, including examples of images that do not contain polyps in the training step, labeling them as background. The dataset was augmented using a series of transformations so that the model would never train twice the exact same image. For each original preprocessed image, an horizontal flip, a vertical flip, and a blur filter have been applied. Thus, we obtain three new images from each original sample. After this data augmentation step, we obtain a dataset that consists of 47.816 images in total (Fig. 12.6).

Our model contains several parameters to be defined in order to improve the results training with some invariant parameters as learning rate 10^{-5}, 1000 iterations per epoch, 32 number of Regional Object Interest (ROIs) and the increased image dataset with rotations and flips. Tests were performed every 50 epochs, selecting different confidence thresholds in order to obtain the best results.

12.3.2 *Neuromation*

In this section, the Neuromation team discusses their model architecture and segmentation uncertainty estimation based on Bayesian approximation.

Network Architecture. The model architecture stems from the Hourglass and U-Net design principles (Ronneberger et al. 2015; Liu et al. 2017). The contracting branch of the model is based on the Resnet-34 encoder where we introduce useful modifications: ELU activations instead of ReLU, reversed order of batch normalization and activation layers (Mishkin et al. 2017), and He normal weight initialization (He et al. 2015). One major difference from the classical U-Net architecture is meant to deal with the limited dataset size characteristic for the GIANA challenge and for medical imaging problems in general. We use two approaches to alleviate the problem of overfitting to limited training data: (1) extreme data augmentation and (2) Spatial 2D Dropout (Tompson et al. 2015) incorporated into the upsampling branch. The upsampling branch is implemented as a Feature Pyramid Network (FPN) (Lin et al. 2016), reconstructing high-level semantic feature maps at 4 scales simultaneously. We implement a Feature Pyramid block as a convolutional layer with 64 activation maps followed by upsampling to the original resolution with upsampling rate of 8, 4, 2, or 1 depending on the feature map depth (see Fig. 12.7). We concatenate upsampled maps into a single layer of $64 \times 4 = 256$ maps and finalize it with the Spatial 2D Dropout layer. Spatial 2D Dropout acts like a regularizer and prevents co-adaptation of the network weights, but unlike conventional dropout it drops out not individual neurons but entire activation maps. In all experiments, we use dropout rate 0.5, i.e., drop 128 out of 256 activation maps.

Finally, the output of the model is a sigmoid layer that assigns to every pixel a continuous probability from 0 to 1 of being a polyp region.

Loss functions. It is known that the categorical cross entropy (CCE), while convenient for training, does not directly translate into the metric of interest, Jaccard index (Rakhlin et al. 2018; Iglovikov et al. 2017; Rakhlin et al. 2019). Hence, as the loss function we use

$$L(w) = (1 - \alpha)CCE(w) - \alpha J(w), \tag{12.1}$$

a weighted sum of CCE and the soft Jaccard loss

$$J = \frac{1}{P}\sum_{p=1}^{P}\left(\frac{y_p \hat{y}_p}{y_p + \hat{y}_p - y_p \hat{y}_p}\right), \tag{12.2}$$

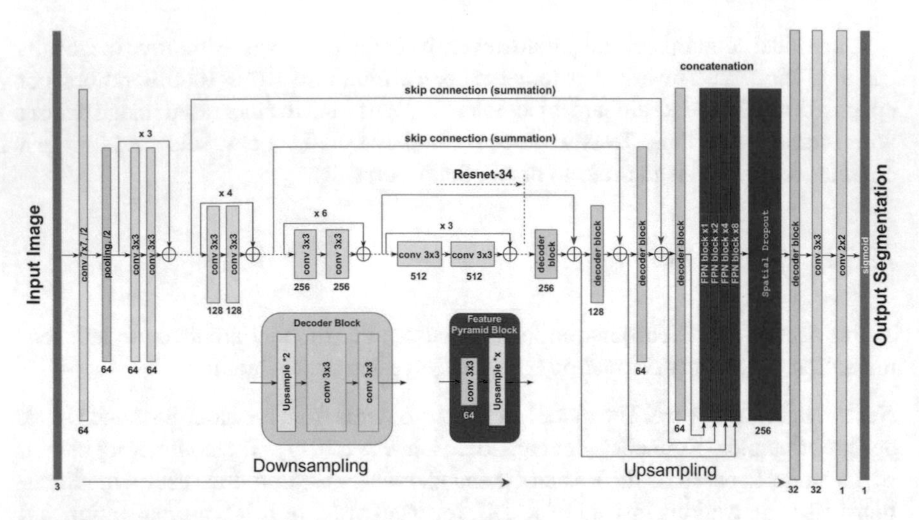

Fig. 12.7 Neuromation architecture

where y_p is the binary label for pixel p, $\hat{y}_p$ is the predicted probability for p, and P is the number of pixels in the image.

Segmentation uncertainty estimation. In the domain of medical imaging, it is particularly important to tell whether a model is confident about its estimate or not. One distinctive feature of our approach is an innovative application of dropout as a Bayesian approximation, as recently proposed by Gal and Ghahramani (2016), http://mlg.eng.cam.ac.uk/yarin/blog_3d801aa532c1ce.html.

Classical deep learning tools do not capture model uncertainty, returning only a point estimate at the output. Using softmax to get probabilities is actually insufficient to obtain model uncertainty (http://mlg.eng.cam.ac.uk/yarin/blog_3d801aa532c1ce.html). Bayesian models, on the other hand, offer a framework suitable to reason about model uncertainty, but usually do it with a prohibitive computational cost. Gal et al. show that dropout neural networks are identical—under certain, not too restrictive, assumptions—to variational inference in Gaussian processes. In particular, they demonstrate "that averaging forward passes through the dropout network is equivalent to Monte Carlo integration over a Gaussian process posterior approximation" (http://mlg.eng.cam.ac.uk/yarin/blog_3d801aa532c1ce.html).

Traditionally, dropout is considered as model averaging, and it was originally explained that scaling the weights at test time without dropout gives a reasonable approximation to the "average" model (Srivastava et al. 2014). However, for convolutional networks this approximation is not sufficient and can be improved considerably (Gal and Ghahramani 2016).

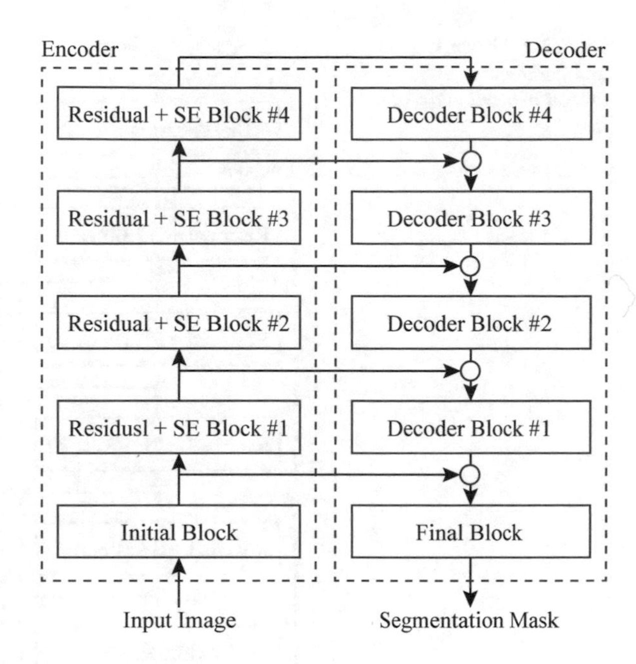

Fig. 12.8 Basic network architecture

12.3.3 *Konica Minolta*

Figure 12.8 shows the basic structure of our network. We use U-Net (Ronneberger et al. 2015) or Link Net (Chaurasia and Culurciello 2017) type deep neural networks with different encoders from the original U-Net and Link Net. U-Net and Link Net both have an encoder-decoder structure and intermediate feature maps in the encoder are concatenated or summed to intermediate feature maps in the decoder, respectively.

12.3.3.1 Modification of Base Architecture

Polyp detection, localization and segmentation tasks Our encoder is based on 101 layer ResNeXt (Xie et al. 2017) with Squeeze-and-Excitation blocks (Hu et al. 2018). The decoder is almost same as the original U-Net and Link Net networks except the number of feature maps. We use Link Net type for the polyp detection task, and use U-Net type network for the polyp localization and segmetation tasks.

WCE detection and localization tasks Figure 12.9 shows the whole structure of our network for the WCE detection and localization tasks. We use Link Net type for the WCE detection and localization tasks. Our encoder is based on 101 layer ResNeXt (Xie et al. 2017) with Squeeze-and-Excitation blocks (Hu et al. 2018). The decoder is almost same as the original U-Net and Link Net networks except the number of feature maps. We add two fully connected layers on top of the last residual block of the encoder (“Residual + SE Block #4” in Fig. 12.9) and obtain the

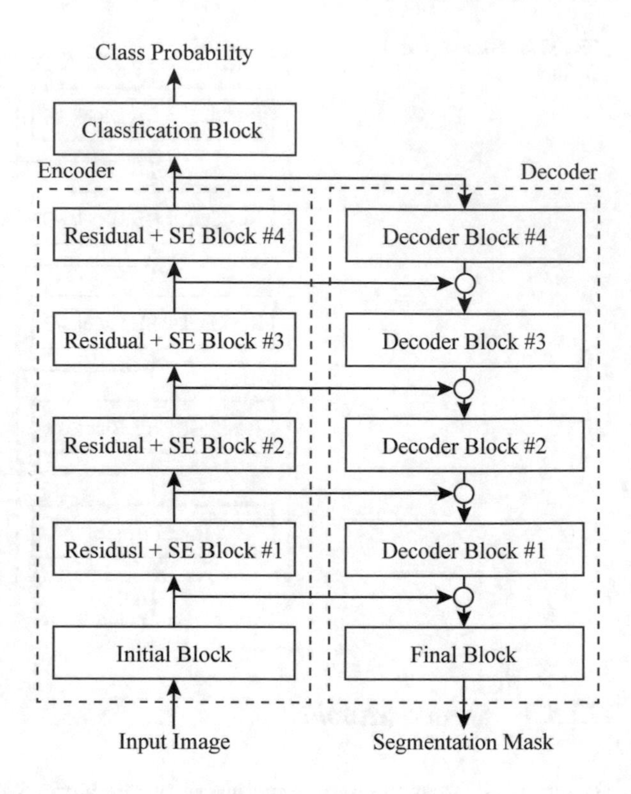

Fig. 12.9 Network architecture for WCE detection and localization task

classification results. We also obtain the lesion area (segmentation mask) as output of the decoder. The network is trained on the tasks of classification and segmentation simultaneously. The locations of the lesions are obtained by post-processing the segmentation results as described later.

12.3.3.2 Parameter Tuning to Solve the Task

Polyp detection, localization and segmentation tasks The training procedure is as follows. An input image is resized to 320 × 320 pixels after the border area is cropped. We use stochastic gradient descent for the optimization. The hyper-parameters in the optimization are that the initial learning rate is 0.1 and the momentum is 0.9. We decay the learning rate with a cosine annealing for each epoch. The mini-batch size is 32 and we run 200 epochs. The loss function is summation of softmax cross entropy loss and dice loss (Milletari et al. 2016). The softmax cross entropy loss is weighted depending on the distance from the contour of the polyp area (Anas et al. 2017). Data augmentation is applied on the fly during the training. We augment using translation, rotation, resizing, flipping, and contrast. We also use mixup (Zhang et al. 2017).

At inference, the final probability map is resized to the original size and thresholded. When probabilities of any pixels are greater than the threshold, we decide there are polyps. Otherwise, we decide there are no polyps.

In the polyp detection task, the threshold value is 0.2 which is decided by using the validation dataset.

In the polyp localization task, the threshold value is 0.4 which is decided by using the validation dataset. When we decide there are polyps, we find the largest area and we use the center of gravity of the largest area as the location of the polyp.

In the polyp segmentation task, the threshold value is 0.3 which is decided by using the validation dataset.

WCE detection and localization tasks The training procedure is as follows. An input image is resized to 320 $\times$ 320 pixels after the border area is cropped. We use stochastic gradient descent for the optimization. The hyper-parameters in the optimization are that the initial learning rate is 0.1 and the momentum is 0.9. We decay the learning rate with a cosine annealing for each epoch. The mini-batch size is 64 and we run 400 epochs. The loss function is summation of the classification loss and the segmentation loss. The classification loss is softmax cross entropy, and the segmentation loss is the summation of pixel-wise softmax cross entropy loss and dice loss (Milletari et al. 2016). Data augmentation is applied on the fly during the training. We augment using translation, rotation, resizing, flipping, and contrast adaptations.

At inference, the classification results are obtained from the output of the fully connected layer on top of the encoder. When the classification result is vascular or inflammatory, we identify the locations of the lesions by using the segmentation result. The segmentation result is obtained from the output of the decoder as a probability map. The probability map is resized to the original image size. Candidates of lesions are regions where the probability is greater than a threshold. If the region size is greater than another threshold, we identify the region as a lesion. The centroids of the detected lesion regions are used as localization results. The threshold values for the probability map and the region size are 0.7 and 50, respectively, which are chosen based on the results on the validation dataset.

12.4 Examples of Results (on the Training Sets)

12.4.1 RTC-ATC

Different experiments were carried out to determine if polyps were detected correctly or not. Tests were performed every 50 epochs, selecting different confidence thresholds in order to obtain the best results. Polyps detection performance is reported in Table 12.1. The results show the robustness of the proposed Faster R-CNN architecture on detecting the polyp position in colonoscopy images with a precision of

Table 12.1 Polyps detection performance. TP: True Positive, FP: False Positive, TN: True Negative, FN: False Negative

TP	FP	TN	FN	Precision	Recall	Accuracy	Specificity	F1	F2
3533	866	1659	1154	80.31	75.37	71.99	65.70	77.76	76.30

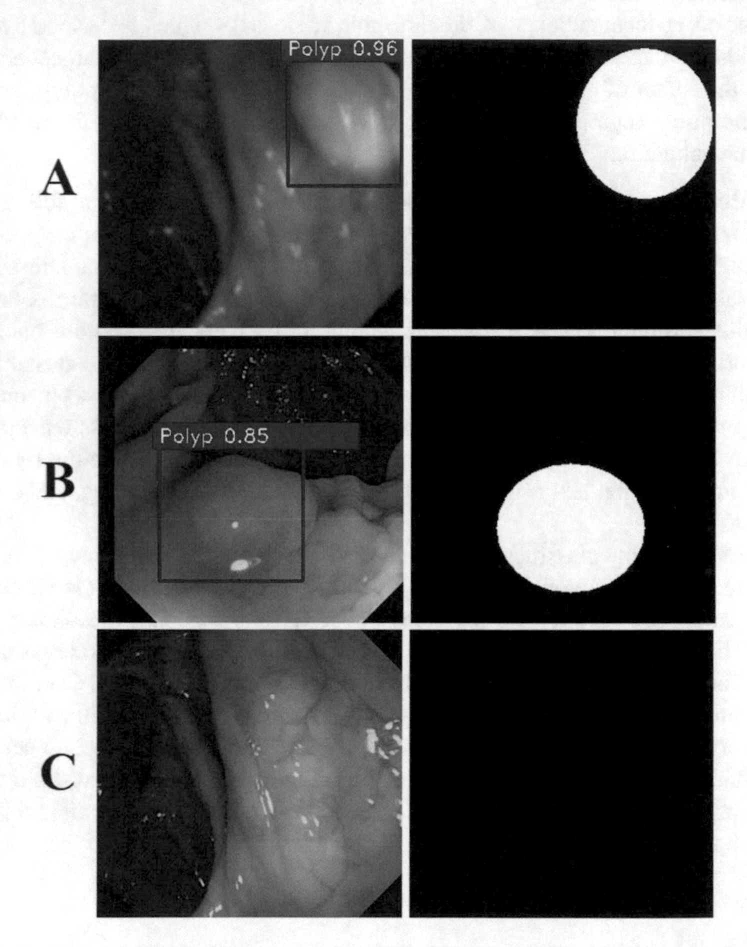

Fig. 12.10 RTC-ATC Polyp detection results task. Left: polyps detected by Faster R-CNN. Confidence values are represented in blue. Right: their corresponding ground truth. A and B show the performance in case a polyp appears, while C shows the performance in case there is no polyp

80.31%, a recall of 75.37%, an accuracy of 71.99% and a specificity of 65.70%. The minimal threshold was established at 0.80.

In Fig. 12.10 the results of our recognition system can be seen by showing the precision when detecting polyps inside samples from the dataset, and their corresponding mask images (as a ground truth) indicating where the polyps are located.

12.4.2 *Neuromation*

A direct application of Gal and Ghahramani (2016), http://mlg.eng.cam.ac.uk/yarin/blog_3d801aa532c1ce.html theory gives us tools to model uncertainty out of deep learning networks at almost zero additional cost. To this end, at test time we do not scale the weights, as it would be in the case of classical dropout. Instead, the model keeps dropping out random activation maps, producing multiple predictions for the same input. This output distribution provides more accurate point estimate and makes possible to assess the uncertainty of polyp segmentation.

Figure 12.11 shows sample segmentation results of our model on validation set samples that we set aside from the training set. It shows, left to right, the original image, ground truth segmentation mask, the model's binary prediction, and, finally, the level of uncertainty estimated by spatial 2D dropout. We see that not only the model shows excellent segmentation results but also assigns reasonable uncertainty values, usually being least certain near the boundaries of a polyp.

12.4.3 *Konica Minolta*

WCE detection and localization tasks We evaluated our proposed method by using the training data set provided in WCE lesion detection and localization challenge in gastrointestinal image analysis (GIANA). The training data set is composed of 600 images without lesion, i.e., normal, 600 images with a vascular lesion and 600 images with an inflammatory lesion. The evaluation was conducted with cross-validation of the training data set. We divided the training data set into six groups and used four groups for training, one group for validation, and one group for testing. Thus, we had six folds for cross-validation and the performance was evaluated with average values and standard deviations of test data in six folds.

We used some evaluation metrics based on the definition in the WCE lesion detection and localization challenge. For classification, we calculated the following metrics; true positive rate (TPR), false positive rate (FPR), false negative rate (FNR), true negative rate (TNR), and accuracy. With respect to localization, we calculated precision, recall, F1 and F2 for two lesion types, i.e., vascular and inflammatory lesions.

Tables 12.2 and 12.3 show the summary of classification and localization performance, respectively. In those tables, the numbers mean "average $\pm$ standard deviation" and the units are percent. The average and standard deviation are calculated for test data of all folds in all lesion types for classification and two lesion types (vascular and inflammatory) for localization.

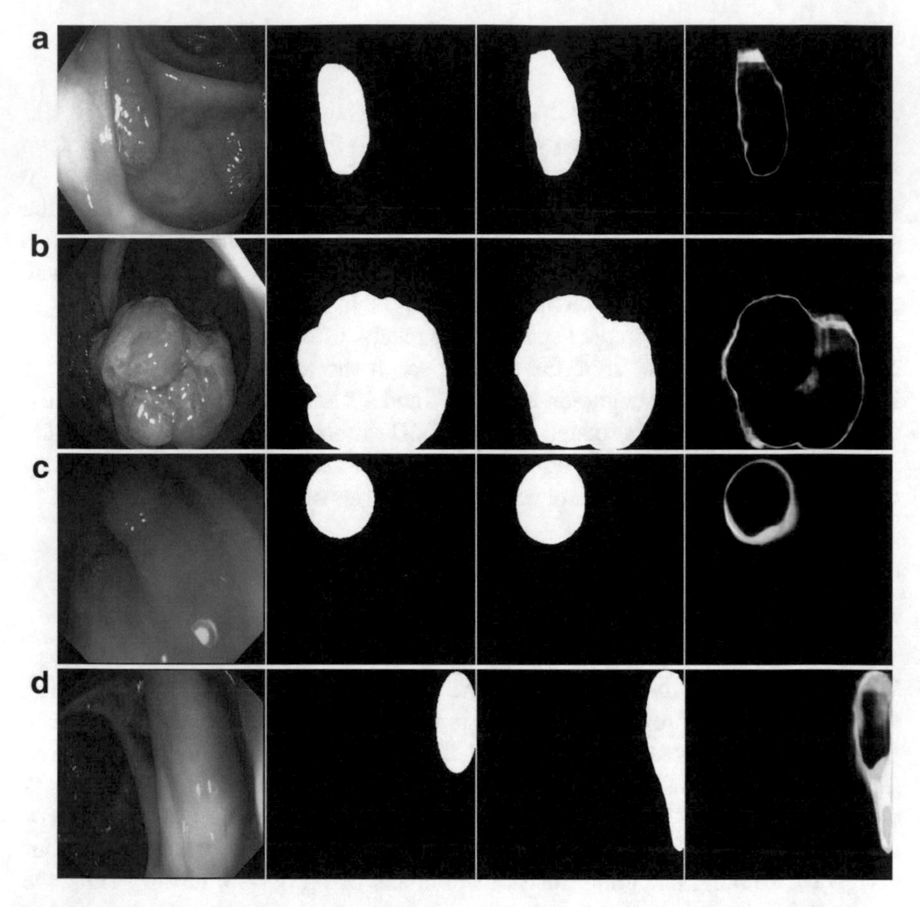

Fig. 12.11 Neuromation results. Left to right: **a** original image, **b** ground truth, **c** predicted mask, **d** uncertainty of the prediction

Table 12.2 Results of classification task

TPR	FPR	FNR	TNR	Accuracy
98.67 ± 0.42	0.67 ± 0.21	1.33 ± 0.42	99.33 ± 0.21	99.11 ± 0.28

Table 12.3 Results of localization task

Precision	Recall	F1	F2
88.76 ± 1.59	76.26 ± 4.05	81.98 ± 2.28	78.44 ± 3.37

References

Anas, E. M. A., Nouranian, S., Mahdavi, S. S., Spadinger, I., Morris, W. J., Salcudean, S. E., Mousavi, P., & Abolmaesumi, P. (2017). Clinical target-volume delineation in prostate brachytherapy using residual neural networks. In *International Conference on Medical Image Computing and Computer-Assisted Intervention* (pp. 365–373). Springer.

Chaurasia, A., & Culurciello, E. (2017). Linknet: Exploiting encoder representations for efficient semantic segmentation. In *2017 IEEE Visual Communications and Image Processing (VCIP)* (pp. 1–4). IEEE.

Felzenszwalb, P. F., Girshick, R. B., McAllester, D., & Ramanan, D. (2009). Object detection with discriminatively trained part-based models. *IEEE Transactions on Pattern Analysis and Machine Intelligence*, *32*(9), 1627–1645.

Gal, Y., & Ghahramani, Z. (2016). Dropout as a Bayesian approximation: Representing model uncertainty in deep learning. In *Proceedings of the 33rd International Conference on Machine Learning (ICML-16)*.

He, K., Zhang, X., Ren, S., & Sun, J. (2015). Delving deep into rectifiers: Surpassing human-level performance on imagenet classification. In *Proceedings of the IEEE International Conference on Computer Vision* (pp. 1026–1034).

He, K., Zhang, X., Ren, S., & Sun, J. (2016). Deep residual learning for image recognition. In *Proceedings of the IEEE Conference on Computer Vision and Pattern Recognition* (pp. 770–778).

Hoang Ngan Le, T., Zheng, Y., Zhu, C., Luu, K., & Savvides, M. (2016). Multiple scale faster-rcnn approach to driver's cell-phone usage and hands on steering wheel detection. In *Proceedings of the IEEE Conference on Computer Vision and Pattern Recognition Workshops* (pp. 46–53).

Hochreiter, S. (1998). The vanishing gradient problem during learning recurrent neural nets and problem solutions. *International Journal of Uncertainty, Fuzziness and Knowledge-Based Systems*, *6*(02), 107–116.

Hu, J., Shen, L., & Sun, G. (2018). Squeeze-and-excitation networks. In *Proceedings of the IEEE Conference on Computer Vision and Pattern Recognition* (pp. 7132–7141).

Iglovikov, V., Rakhlin, A., Kalinin, A., & Shvets, A. (2017). Pediatric bone age assessment using deep convolutional neural networks. arXiv preprint arXiv:1712.05053.

Jiang, H., & Learned-Miller, E. (2017). Face detection with the faster r-cnn. In *2017 12th IEEE International Conference on Automatic Face & Gesture Recognition (FG 2017)* (pp. 650–657). IEEE.

Lin, T., Dollár, P., Girshick, R. B., He, K., Hariharan, B., & Belongie, S. J. (2016). Feature pyramid networks for object detection. *CoRR*, arXiv:abs/1612.03144.

Liu, Y., Minh Nguyen, D., Deligiannis, N., Ding, W., & Munteanu, A. (2017). Hourglass-shapenetwork based semantic segmentation for high resolution aerial imagery. *Remote Sensing* (vol. 9(6), p. 522).

Milletari, F., Navab, N., & Ahmadi, S.-A. (2016). V-net: Fully convolutional neural networks for volumetric medical image segmentation. In *2016 Fourth International Conference on 3D Vision (3DV)* (pp. 565–571). IEEE.

Mishkin, D., Sergievskiy, N., & Matas, J. (2017). Systematic evaluation of convolution neural network advances on the imagenet. *Computer Vision and Image Understanding*.

Rakhlin, A., Davydow, A., & Nikolenko, S. (2018, June). Land cover classification from satellite imagery with u-net and lovász-softmax loss. In *The IEEE Conference on Computer Vision and Pattern Recognition (CVPR) Workshops*, June 2018.

Rakhlin, A., Tiulpin, A., Shvets, A. A., Kalinin, A. A., Iglovikov, V. I., & Nikolenko, S. (2019). Breast tumor cellularity assessment using deep neural networks. In *The IEEE International Conference on Computer Vision (ICCV) Workshops*, Oct 2019.

Ren, S., He, K., Girshick, R., & Sun, J. (2015). Faster r-cnn: Towards real-time object detection with region proposal networks. In *Advances in neural information processing systems* (pp. 91–99).

Ronneberger, O., Fischer, P., & Brox, T. (2015). U-net: Convolutional networks for biomedical image segmentation. In *International Conference on Medical Image Computing and Computer-Assisted Intervention* (pp. 234–241). Springer.

Srivastava, N., Hinton, G., Krizhevsky, A., Sutskever, I., & Salakhutdinov, R. (2014). Dropout: A simple way to prevent neural networks from overfitting. *Journal of Machine Learning Research, 15*, 1929–1958.

Tompson, J., Goroshin, R., Jain, A., LeCun, Y., & Bregler, C. (2015). Efficient object localization using convolutional networks. In *Proceedings of the IEEE Conference on Computer Vision and Pattern Recognition* (pp. 648–656).

"What My Deep Model Doesn't Know...." http://mlg.eng.cam.ac.uk/yarin/blog_3d801aa532c1ce.html.

Xie, S., Girshick, R., Dollár, P., Tu, Z., & He, K. (2017). Aggregated residual transformations for deep neural networks. In *Proceedings of the IEEE Conference on Computer Vision and Pattern Recognition* (pp. 1492–1500).

Zhang, H., Cisse, M., Dauphin, Y. N., & Lopez-Paz, D. (2017). mixup: Beyond empirical risk minimization. arXiv preprint arXiv:1710.09412.

Chapter 13
Multi-scale Ensemble of ResNet Variants

Joost van der Putten and Farhad Ghazvinian Zanjani

13.1 Motivation

Residual learning has become a staple in the deep learning community due to its simple yet effective design. ResNets have been successfully employed for a variety of problems (Tan et al. 2018; Chen et al. 2018; Habibzadeh et al. 2018; Putten et al. 2019). Additionally, we incorporate multi-scale information in our approach by training models with different input image resolutions. This approach is taken since multi-scale approaches have been shown to be effective for many medical image analysis problems (Litjens et al. 2017). Finally, ensembling is a good way to boost performance and ensembles have been used to win many AI competitions. These methods are especially effective when the models are diverse (Brown et al. 2005). We achieve this diversity by using different ResNet models and by employing the multi-scale approach.

13.2 Methods

13.2.1 Pre-processing

All images are pre-processed before the actual training process. A few images had a larger resolution of 704×704 pixels, these instances were first resized to 576×576 pixels in order to keep the images on the same scale. Second, the black borders surrounding the endoscopic field of view were also removed before training. This was done for two reasons: (1) it removes redundant useless information and (2)

J. van der Putten (✉) · F. G. Zanjani
Eindhoven University of Technology, VCA Group, TU/e-VCA, Den Dolech 2, 5600 MB Eindhoven, The Netherlands
e-mail: j.a.v.d.putten@tue.nl

J. Bernal and A. Histace (eds.), *Computer-Aided Analysis of Gastrointestinal Videos*,
https://doi.org/10.1007/978-3-030-64340-9_13

timestamps in the corners of the images could cause an unwanted bias. The image resolution after pre-processing is 512 × 512 × 3 for all images in the data set.

13.2.2 Class Split

The classification process was split up into two binary classification problems instead of one ternary problem. First, we train a network to classify the images as either normal or diseased frames (Vascular Lesion (VL) and Inflammatory Lesion (IL) combined), with a training set which contains 600 normal images and 1212 diseased images. Second, we train a separate network to classify the diseased images as either VL or IL, with a training set of 605 vascular lesions and 607 inflammatory lesions. This approach was taken as initial experiments showed poor results on the ternary problem. By simplifying the difficult ternary problem into two easier binary problems, the validation results were increased substantially.

13.2.3 Training Details

13.2.3.1 Transfer Learning

For the normal-diseased classification we use several models pre-trained on ImageNet (Deng et al. 2009). We employed several versions of the widely used ResNet architecture for our approach. Table 13.1 shows all ResNet (He et al. 2016) variants that were used for this solution. ResNet like architectures have become a staple in deep learning since the introduction in 2016 (Tan et al. 2018). Many works have successfully used networks with residual connections such as in road scene segmentation (Chen et al. 2018), or white blood cell classification (Habibzadeh et al. 2018). Residual Networks have also been successfully used for artificial intelligence in endoscopy (Putten et al. 2019). In this work, we employ fully convolutional versions of these networks, so we have no restrictions on the input dimensions of the networks. This facilitates the training of 3 separate models for each of the architectures in Table 13.1, the first with the original input resolution (512 × 512), the second where the input resolution is resized to 256 × 256 pixels and a third where we resize the images to 128 × 128 pixels. This approach results in 15 trained networks for the classification of normal images versus diseased images that operate on different scales. This multi-scale approach is also commonly used in medical imaging analysis (Litjens et al. 2017). More information on the combination of these models is further described in Sect. 13.2.4.

The same approach is taken for the vascular lesion versus inflammatory lesion classification with one difference. Instead of using networks pre-trained on ImageNet, we use the weights of the networks obtained in the normal-diseased classification stage.

Table 13.1 Base architecures used for this solution

Model	Description
ResNet18	ResNet architecture with 18 convolutional layers
ResNet34	ResNet architecture with 34 convolutional layers
ResNet50	ResNet architecture with 50 convolutional layers
ResNet101	ResNet architecture with 101 convolutional layers
ResNext (Xie et al. 2017)	Adaptation of ResNet where each Residual block is split up into a large amount of 3×3 convolutions after applying a bottleneck layer

13.2.3.2 Two-stage training

In order to fully leverage the effectiveness of the transfer learning strategy, we train our model in two stages. First, as we need to replace the final layer to suit our binary classification problem, the corresponding weights are not yet trained in the normal-diseased classification part. For that reason, all weights of the model are frozen except for the final layer and are trained for one epoch with a starting learning rate (λ) of 10 ^{2}, for the rest of the epoch we decay λ with cosine annealing every batch in such a way that the learning rate equals 10^{-4} at the end of the epoch. During the disease-classification part, this first step is skipped as we already have a binary output. The learning rates for all models were obtained with the learning rate range test.

We use differential learning rates in the second stage of training. Differential learning rates capitalize on the tendency of neural nets to learn basic features such as edges and shapes in the first few layers, and complex features such as, in the case of ImageNet, faces, and dog breeds. We assume the former are still very useful for our goal while the later are nearly useless. First, we unfreeze all weights of the model. Second, the learning rates for the layers are changed depending on depth. λ of the final third are set to 10^{-2}. Maximum λ of the middle third of the layers and first third of the layers are set to 5^{-3} and 10^{-3}, respectively. This approach allows the optimizer to update the weights in the later irrelevant layers more aggressively than in the early layers containing relevant low-level features. We train the model for five cycles with a cyclical learning rate scheduler (Smith 2017) and a cycle multiplier of 2.

13.2.4 Ensembling

After training all models, each model's prediction score is saved for each image. Resulting in 15 classification scores per image. These scores are then fed into a final fully connected neural network with only one hidden layer and 20 hidden neurons. The output of this model is a binary classification (normal-disease or VL-IL). This small network automatically learns which of the 15 models contribute the most to the final classification. One ensemble network is trained for each of the classification

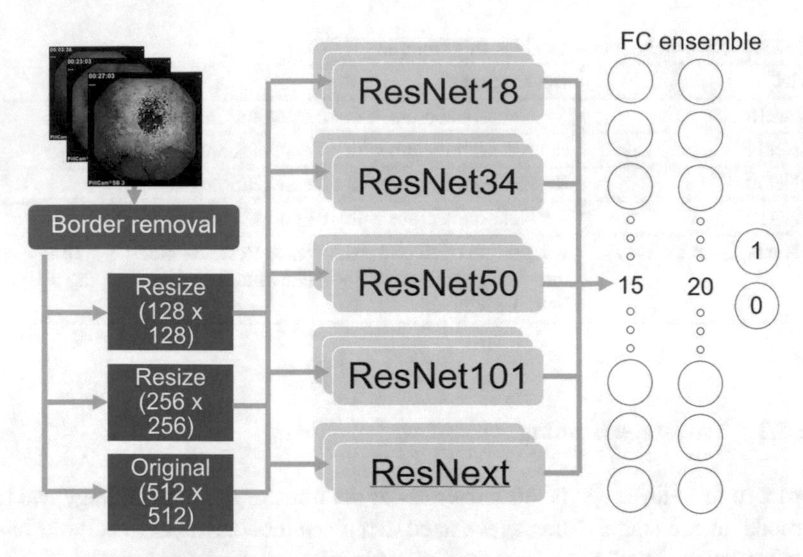

Fig. 13.1 Schematic overview of the used models and the ensembling method. A given input image is fed to five different models with three different input resolutions. The outputs of the resulting 15 models are then finally fed to a small fully connected network to determine a final classification label

parts. Ensembling almost always improves classification performance compared to singe model predictions. When there is no limitation on the amount of available compute, ensembling is a good way to boost performance (Dietterich 2000). An overview of the used model is shown in Fig. 13.1.

13.2.5 Test-Time Augmentation

At test time, we predict the probability that a certain patch belongs to a class as usual. In addition to that we also predict the class of eight random transformations of the same image. The transformations used in this case are the same transformations used as data augmentation during training. In this work we use random flipping (horizontal and vertical), random zoom with a maximum zoom of 10%, and balance and contrast adjustments. This results in nine classification probabilities of slight permutations of the same image. The average of these predictions is in many cases a better class indicator than using only the original image.

13.2.6 Validation

To determine hyper parameters such as learning rate, batch size, and stopping criteria, 25% of the training set is randomly selected to validate the model. After determining the optimal hyperparameter settings, the entire model is retrained with all available labeled data using the optimal hyperparameters. Then, the entire test set is first classified into diseased versus normal with the first model. Finally, the samples classified as diseased are further split into vascular lesion or inflammatory lesion with the second model.

References

Brown, G., Wyatt, J., Harris, R., & Yao, X. (2005). Diversity creation methods: A survey and categorisation. *Information Fusion, 6*(1), 5–20.

Chen, L.-C., Zhu, Y., Papandreou, G., Schroff, F., & Adam, H. (2018). Encoder-decoder with atrous separable convolution for semantic image segmentation. In *Proceedings of the European Conference on Computer Vision (ECCV)* (pp. 801–818).

Deng, J., Dong, W., Socher, R., Li, L.-J., Li, K., & Fei-Fei, L. (2009). Imagenet: A large-scale hierarchical image database. In *2009 IEEE Conference on Computer Vision and Pattern Recognition* (pp. 248–255). IEEE.

Dietterich, T. G. (2000). Ensemble methods in machine learning. In *International Workshop on Multiple Classifier Systems* (pp. 1–15). Springer.

Habibzadeh, M., Jannesari, M., Rezaei, Z., Baharvand, H., & Totonchi, M. (2018). Automatic white blood cell classification using pre-trained deep learning models: Resnet and inception. In *Tenth International Conference on Machine Vision (ICMV 2017)* (Vol. 10696, p. 1069612). International Society for Optics and Photonics.

He, K., Zhang, X., Ren, S., & Sun, J. (2016). Deep residual learning for image recognition. In *Proceedings of the IEEE Conference on Computer Vision and Pattern Recognition* (pp. 770–778).

Litjens, G., Kooi, T., Bejnordi, B. E., Setio, A. A. A., Ciompi, F., Ghafoorian, M., et al. (2017). A survey on deep learning in medical image analysis. *Medical Image Analysis, 42*, 60–88.

Smith, L. N. (2017). Cyclical learning rates for training neural networks. In *2017 IEEE Winter Conference on Applications of Computer Vision (WACV)* (pp. 464–472). IEEE.

Tan, C., Sun, F., Kong, T., Zhang, W., Yang, Y., Liu, C. (2018). A survey on deep transfer learning. In *International Conference on Artificial Neural Networks* (pp. 270–279). Springer.

van der Putten, J., de Groof, J., van der Sommen, F., Struyvenberg, M., Zinger, S., Curvers, W., Schoon, E., Bergman, J., et al. (2019). Pseudo-labeled bootstrapping and multi-stage transfer learning for the classification and localization of dysplasia in barrett's esophagus. In *International Workshop on Machine Learning in Medical Imaging* (pp. 169–177). Springer.

Xie, S., Girshick, R., Dollár, P., Tu, Z., & He, K. (2017). Aggregated residual transformations for deep neural networks. In *Proceedings of the IEEE Conference on Computer Vision and Pattern Recognition* (pp. 1492–1500).

Chapter 14
Convolutional LSTM

Tom Eelbode, Pieter Sinonquel, Raf Bisschops, and Frederik Maes

14.1 Introduction

A common limitation to almost all state-of-the-art techniques for automated polyp detection and delineation is that they are based on still-frame analysis (Wang et al. 2018; Urban et al. 2018; Shin et al. 2018; Mohammed et al. 2018). Colonoscopy, however, is a video-based modality and an endoscopist will always use the contextual information from previous frames to make an accurate decision about the potential presence of a polyp. Recent developments in semantic segmentation of videos in non-medical applications (Fayyaz et al. 2016; Valipour et al. 2017) show that including temporal features in a CNN can increase its performance and also yield more consistent results over time. Recurrent neural networks (RNNs) are a commonly used concept for sequence modeling and essentially allow neural networks to retain information over time. Long short-term memory (LSTM) models are a type of RNNs that can model longer time dependencies than traditional RNNs and it is a convolutional variant of these LSTM models (Xingjian et al. 2015) that is used in this chapter. The latter can not only encode temporal features but can simultaneously incorporate spatial features into one single layer.

We extend a state of the art, non-medical object segmentation network—Deeplabv3+ (Chen et al. 2018)—with a convolutional LTSM layer in its decoder. This allows the use of a pretrained network and to finetune it to our relatively small polyps dataset. This makes the training of the LSTM layers much faster and easier to converge.

T. Eelbode (✉) · F. Maes
Medical Imaging Research Center, ESAT/PSI, MIRC, KU Leuven, Herestraat 49 - bus, 7003, 3000 Leuven, Belgium
e-mail: tom.eelbode@kuleuven.be

P. Sinonquel · R. Bisschops
Department of Gastroenterology and Hepatology, UZ Leuven, Herestraat 49, 3000 Leuven, Belgium

J. Bernal and A. Histace (eds.), *Computer-Aided Analysis of Gastrointestinal Videos*,
https://doi.org/10.1007/978-3-030-64340-9_14

14.2 Methods

In this work, an extension to the powerful Deeplab v3+ (Chen et al. 2018) is proposed where a convolutional LSTM layer is introduced at the deepest level as illustrated in Fig. 14.1. Deeplab is an encoder-decoder network that uses spatial pyramid pooling modules for multi-scale contextual information extraction. It effectively models rich semantic information on a coarse level, but also captures fine object details along its boundaries. The former (the coarse features) typically have a more continuous course over sequential frames (Shelhamer et al. 2016) and having access to these features from previous frames might help with segmentation. That's why here, these high-level features are fed to a convLSTM layer before they are up-sampled and concatenated with the low-level features. All layers are identical to the original Deeplab architecture except for this one added layer. This has the advantage that we can use a pretrained encoder. The original model is pretrained on Imagenet and then further finetuned for single frame prediction of colonic polyps before the convLTSM layer is added.

The training of the network is done in three sequential steps:

1. Finetuning of Deeplab on GIANA dataset
   We use the original Deeplabv3+ architecture with Xception backbone pretrained on the PASCAL VOC 2012 challenge dataset (Everingham et al. 2010). This network is then finetuned on the GIANA Challenge dataset by progressively setting more layers as trainable starting from the final layer. We use the Adam optimizer with focal loss (Lin et al. 2017) and a learning rate of $1e^{-5}$ for 1000 epochs. Steps per epoch are 50 steps for a batch size of 16 full images.
2. Changing architecture towards recurrent model
   The Deeplab architecture is extended by introducing the ConvLTSM layer into

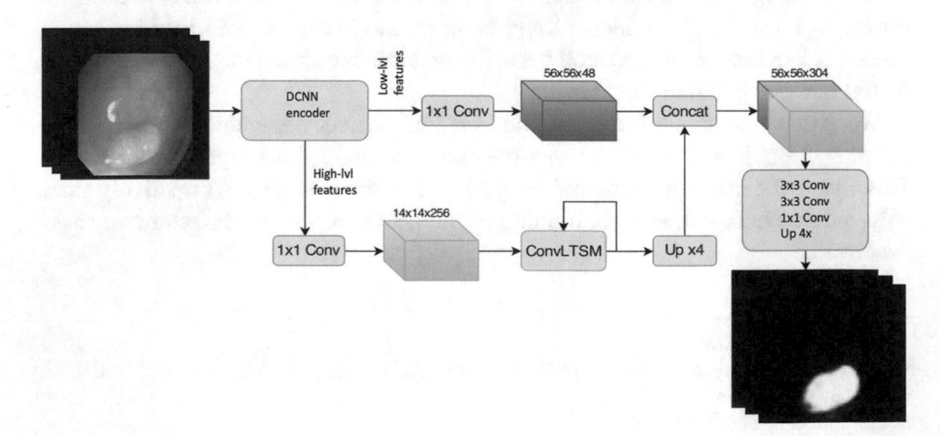

Fig. 14.1 Our proposed extension to Deeplabv3+ places a convLSTM layer after the high-level features are extracted. This gives the decoder network access to relevant semantic information from the previous frames

the decoder. The rest of the architecture is left unaltered such that we can re-use the weights from step 1 for further training. We found that loading weights from the previously trained network allow for a much faster and more robust training of the RNN compared to training it from scratch.

3. Training of Deeplab_rec on GIANA dataset with BPTT
The decoder part of our recurrent deeplab model is retrained with the same dataset as before. To train a recurrent neural network, one cannot simply use backpropagation as for a standard CNN model. In order to also learn temporal dependencies, we use truncated backpropagation through time (BPTT) with 10 timesteps. Once again, we use the Adam optimizer with focal loss and a learning rate of $1e^{-5}$. We train for 30 epochs with 100 steps per epoch and a batch size of 16 sequences.

For training, the oval-shaped CVC_video annotations are used directly for training this dense segmentation network. Although not ideal since edges of the polyps will most likely not be recovered, we see that it can still converge and learn the location of the polyp in this way. During training, intensive data augmentation is used: rotation, flipping, random cropping and width shifting, color and brightness disturbance, and blurring. All experiments were run on a single NVIDIA RTX 2080 Ti GPU card with 11Gb of memory.

14.3 Task-Specific Parameter Tuning

The same method was applied to each of the first four tasks, being polyp detection, localization, segmentation, and HD segmentation. This section describes the differences between the implementations for each task.

14.3.1 Polyp Detection

Pre-processing—The original images of size 384×288 are cropped and subsequently bilinearly downsampled to fit the network's input size of 224×224. Their histograms are equalized with contrast limited adaptive histogram equalization (CLAHE) and they are normalized to zero mean and a variance of 1 on a sample level.
Post-processing—The output of the network is a segmentation map for each image indicating the probability of every pixel belonging to a polyp or not. A simple blob detector is applied to these segmentation maps to identify any coherent blobs with sufficient probability. The center points of these blobs are then used as candidates for possible polyp locations. A confidence score is then calculated for each candidate based on the output probability of the network in that region and also on whether or not the previous frames had a candidate in roughly the same location. This confidence value is then thresholded to determine final polyp locations. The output value for

polyp detection is then determined by the presence in the entire frame of a polyp candidate with a high enough confidence value.

14.3.2 Polyp Localization

The process for this task is completely identical to the one for polyp detection (Sect. 14.3.1). The output is however not just the frame-wide prediction, but each candidate location is returned with its confidence value.

14.3.3 Polyp Segmentation

The data for this task was slightly different. The frames in this dataset were not sequential and an oval-shaped annotated ground truth was provided for each image. Since no temporal information was available, the same network was applied but without the convLSTM layer (i.e., the original Deeplabv3+ model). This model was then also finetuned on the segmentation training set.
Pre-processing—This is almost identical to the process defined for polyp detection in Sect. 14.3.1 except for the resizing. The original images of size 574 × 500 were squashed immediately to fit the network's input dimensions of 224 × 224 without cropping since there was only a small difference in aspect ratio.
Post-processing—The output probability map is passed to a fully connected CRF in order to finetune the predictions to the finer edges (Krähenbühl and Koltun 2011). The resulting probability map is thresholded and any remaining holes are filled.

14.3.4 Polyp Segmentation HD

Pre-processing The process is identical to that for the SD except for one pre-processing step. The black borders on the image are cropped before further processing the image. This way, a large portion of the image (which is not of interest) is removed and the size of the input image is significantly lower. The non-temporal polyp segmentation network from the previous subsection is finetuned once more for these higher resolution images.

In this chapter, a state-of-the-art object segmentation network is extended with a ConvLSTM layer to incorporate temporal features into the decoder of the network. Access to this temporal information has the potential to decreases the number of false positives detected by the network without any decrease in sensitivity. In Eelbode et al. (2019), it is shown that treating colonoscopy as a video-based modality instead of processing each frame individually, is feasible and beneficial in terms of detection performance. Especially for confusing frames (such as blurry or artefact-containing frames), the recurrent version is more robust. The same technique is applied here with a few limitations: the number of polyp sequences to train on in the GIANA dataset is much lower, the nature of the ground truths for these sequences is also less informative since these are bounding boxes as opposed to dense delineations. Additionally, this technique delivers dense segmentations for each frame as opposed to the frame-level classification or location that is needed for the polyp detection and localization task in this challenge. This makes the post-processing a vital step for the result and effectively makes the model not end-to-end trainable for this task. The segmentation task on the other hand does expect these dense outputs, but there is no temporal information available for these subtasks. The full benefit of this method should therefore be evaluated on a different type of dataset which will hopefully be available in future GIANA challenge editions.

In future work, we will investigate how this technique can be extended for video-based polyp characterization, i.e., the automated identification of the polyp type (malignant or benign). We believe that for this type of application, inclusion of temporal information will be even more important since an endoscopist also needs to inspect a polyp from multiple angles to make an accurate prediction of its type.

References

Chen, L.-C., et al. (2018). Encoder-decoder with atrous separable convolution for semantic image segmentation. arXiv preprint arXiv:1802.02611.

Chen, L.-C., Zhu, Y., Papandreou, G., Schroff, F., & Adam, H. (2018). Encoder-decoder with atrous separable convolution for semantic image segmentation. arXiv preprint arXiv:1802.02611.

Eelbode, T., Demedts, I., Bisschops, R., Roelandt, P., Hassan, C., Coron, E., Bhandari, P., Neumann, H., Pech, O., Repici, A., et al. (2019). Tu1931 incorporation of temporal information in a deep neural network improves performance level for automated polyp detection and delineation. *Gastrointestinal Endoscopy*, *89*(6), AB618–AB619.

Everingham, M., Van Gool, L., Williams, C. K. I., Winn, J., Zisserman, A., Everingham, M., Van Gool Leuven, L. K., CKI Williams, B., Winn, J., & Zisserman, A. (2010). The PASCAL visual object classes (VOC) challenge. *International Journal of Computer Vision*, *88*, 303–338.

Fayyaz, M., et al. (2016). Stfcn: Spatio-temporal fcn for semantic video segmentation. arXiv preprint arXiv:1608.05971.

Krähenbühl, P., & Koltun, V. (2011). Efficient inference in fully connected crfs with gaussian edge potentials. In *Advances in neural information processing systems* (pp. 109–117).

Lin, T.-Y., Goyal, P., Girshick, R., He, K., & Dollár, P. (2017). Focal loss for dense object detection. In *Proceedings of the IEEE International Conference on Computer Vision* (pp. 2980–2988).

Mohammed, A., Yildirim, S., Farup, I., Pedersen, M., & Hovde, Ø. (2018). Y-net: A deep convolutional neural network for polyp detection. arXiv preprint arXiv:1806.01907.

Shelhamer, E., Rakelly, K., Hoffman, J., & Darrell, T. (2016). Clockwork convnets for video semantic segmentation. In *European Conference on Computer Vision* (pp. 852–868). Springer.

Shin, Y., Qadir, H. A., Aabakken, L., Bergsland, J., & Balasingham, I. (2018). Automatic colon polyp detection using region based deep CNN and post learning approaches. *IEEE Access*, *6*, 40950–40962.

Urban, G., Tripathi, P., Alkayali, T., Mittal, M., Jalali, F., Karnes, W., et al. (2018). Deep learning localizes and identifies polyps in real time with 96% accuracy in screening colonoscopy. *Gastroenterology*, *155*(4), 1069–1078.e8.

Valipour, S., Siam, M., Jagersand, M., & Ray, N. (2017). Recurrent fully convolutional networks for video segmentation. In *2017 IEEE Winter Conference on Applications of Computer Vision (WACV)* (pp. 29–36). IEEE.

Wang, P., Xiao, X., Glissen Brown, J. R., Berzin, T. M., Tu, M., Xiong, F., Hu, X., Liu, P., Song, Y., Zhang, D., Yang, X., Li, L., He, J., Yi, X., Liu, J., & Liu, X. (2018). Development and validation of a deep-learning algorithm for the detection of polyps during colonoscopy. *Nature Biomedical Engineering*, *2*(10), 741–748.

Xingjian, S., Chen, Z., Wang, H., Yeung, D.-Y., Wong, W.-K., & Woo, W.-c. (2015). Convolutional LSTM network: A machine learning approach for precipitation nowcasting. In *Advances in neural information processing systems* (pp. 802–810).

Chapter 15
TernausNet

Vladimir I. Iglovikov and Alexey A. Shvets

15.1 Model Architecture

In this work we evaluate four different deep architectures for segmentation: U-Net (Ronneberger et al. 2015), two modifications of TernausNet (Iglovikov and Shvets 2018), and a modification of LinkNet called AlbuNet34 (Chaurasia and Culurciello 2017; Shvets et al. 2018).

In general, a U-Net-like architecture consists of a contracting path to capture context and of a symmetrically expanding path that enables precise localization (for example, see Fig. 15.1). The contracting path follows the typical architecture of a convolutional network with alternating convolution and pooling operations and progressively downsamples feature maps, increasing the number of feature maps per layer at the same time. Every step in the expansive path consists of an upsampling of the feature map followed by a convolution. Hence, the expansive branch increases the resolution of the output. In order to localize, upsampled features, the expansive path combines them with high-resolution features from the contracting path via skip-connections (Ronneberger et al. 2015). The output of the model is a pixel-by-pixel mask that shows the class of each pixel. We use slightly modified version of the original U-Net model that previously proved itself very useful for segmentation problems with limited amounts of data, for example, see (Iglovikov et al. 2018). Our submission to the MICCAI 2017 Endoscopic Vision SubChallenge: Angiodysplasia detection and localization is produced using this architecture.

As an improvement over the standard U-Net architecture, we use similar networks with pre-trained encoders. TernausNet (Iglovikov and Shvets 2018) is a U-Net-like

V. I. Iglovikov
ODS.ai, San Francisco, USA
e-mail: iglovikov@gmail.com

A. A. Shvets (✉)
Massachusetts Institute of Technology - MIT, Cambridge, USA
e-mail: shvets@mit.edu

J. Bernal and A. Histace (eds.), *Computer-Aided Analysis of Gastrointestinal Videos*,
https://doi.org/10.1007/978-3-030-64340-9_15

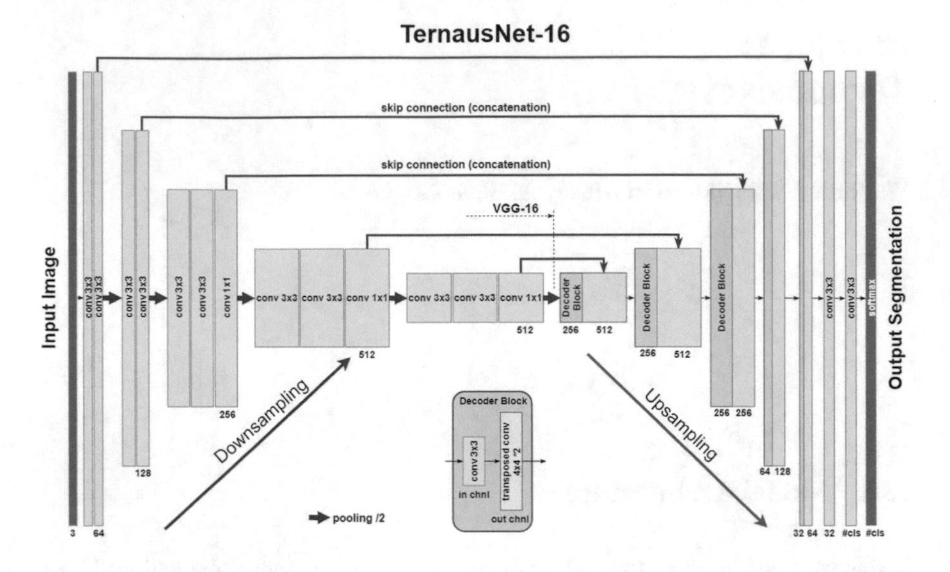

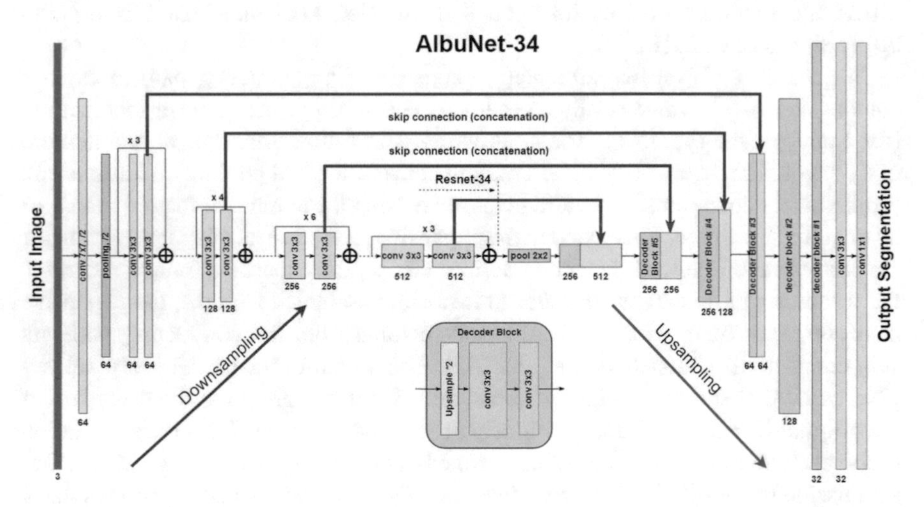

Fig. 15.1 These segmentation networks are based on encoder-decoder network of U-Net family. TernausNet uses pre-trained VGG16 network as an encoder, while AlbuNet34 uses pre-trained ResNet34 as an encoder. It is different from TernausNet in that it adds skip-connections to the upsampling path, while TernausNet concatenates downsampled layers with the upsampling path (just like original U-Net does). Each box corresponds to a multi-channel feature map. The number of channels is pointed below the box. The height of the box represents a feature map resolution. The blue arrows denote skip-connections where information is transmitted from the encoder to the decoder

architecture that uses relatively simple pre-trained VGG11 or VGG16 (Simonyan and Zisserman 2014) networks as an encoder (see Fig. 15.1). VGG11 consists of seven convolutional layers, each followed by a ReLU activation function, and five max polling operations, each reducing feature map by 2. All convolutional layers have 3×3 kernels. TernausNet16 has a similar structure and uses VGG16 network as an encoder (see Fig. 15.1).

In contrast, AlbuNet uses an encoder based on a ResNet-type architecture (He et al. 2016). In this work, we use pre-trained ResNet34, see Fig. 15.1. The encoder starts with the initial block that performs convolution with a kernel of size 7×7 and stride 2. This block is followed by max-pooling with stride 2. The later portion of the network consists of repetitive residual blocks. In every residual block, the first convolution operation is implemented with stride 2 to provide downsampling, while the rest convolution operations use stride 1. In addition, the decoder of the network consists of several decoder blocks that are connected with the corresponding encoder block. As for TernausNets, the transmitted block from the encoder is concatenated to the corresponding decoder block. Each decoder block includes 1×1 convolution operation that reduces the number of filters by 4, followed by batch normalization and transposed convolution to upsample the feature map.

15.2 Model Training

We use Jaccard index (Intersection Over Union) as the evaluation metric. It can be interpreted as a similarity measure between a finite number of sets. For two sets A and B, it can be defined as following:

$$J(A, B) = \frac{|A \cap B|}{|A \cup B|} = \frac{|A \cap B|}{|A| + |B| - |A \cap B|} \tag{15.1}$$

Since an image consists of pixels, the last expression can be adapted for discrete objects in the following way:

$$J = \frac{1}{n} \sum_{i=1}^{n} \left(\frac{y_i \hat{y}_i}{y_i + \hat{y}_i - y_i \hat{y}_i} \right) \tag{15.2}$$

where y_i and $\hat{y}_i$ are a binary value (label) and a predicted probability for the pixel i, correspondingly.

Since image segmentation task can also be considered as a pixel classification problem, we additionally use common classification loss functions, denoted as H in 15.3. For a the binary segmentation problem H is a binary cross entropy, while for the multi-class segmentation problem H is a categorical cross entropy.

The final expression for the generalized loss function is obtained by combining (15.2) and H as following:

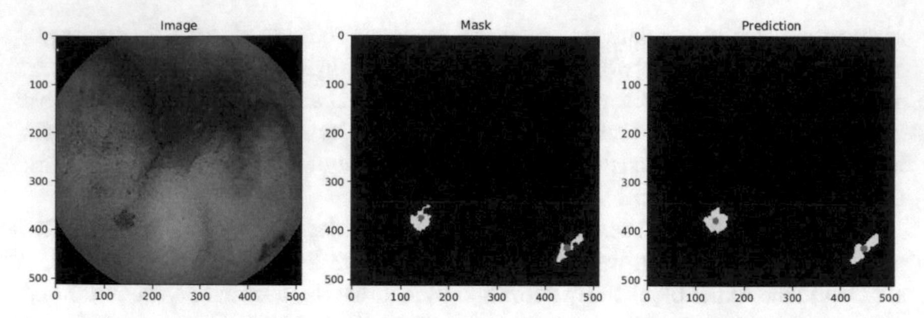

Fig. 15.2 The prediction of our detector on the validation set image. Here, the left panel shows the original image, the middle panel shows the ground truth training mask, and the right panel shows the predicted mask. Green dots inside of each mask corresponds to the centroid that defines angiodysplasia localization output. Here, for example, the real and predicted values for centroid coordinates correspondingly are $p^1_{mask} = (376, 144)$, $p^1_{pred} = (380, 143)$ for the first mask and $p^2_{mask} = (437, 445)$, $p^2_{pred} = (437, 447)$ for the second mask

$$L = H - \log J \tag{15.3}$$

By minimizing this loss function, we simultaneously maximize probabilities for correct pixels to be predicted and maximize the intersection J between masks and corresponding predictions, which improves overall segmentation performance (Iglovikov and Shvets 2018). Each model is trained with Adam optimizer for 10 epochs with learning rate 0.001, and then for another 5 epochs with the learning rate 0.0001.

15.3 Postprocessing

At the output of a model, we obtain an image, in which each pixel value corresponds to a probability of belonging to the area of interest or a class. The size of the output image matches the input image size. For binary segmentation, we use 0.3 as a threshold value (chosen using validation dataset) to binarize pixel probabilities. All pixel values below the specified threshold are set to 0, while all values above the threshold are set to 255 to produce final prediction mask.

Following the segmentation step, we perform postprocessing in order to find the coordinates of angiodysplasia lesions in the image. In the postprocessing step we use OpenCV implementation of connected component labeling function: `connectedComponentsWithStats`. This function returns the number of connected components, their sizes (areas), and centroid coordinates of the corresponding connected component. In our detector we use another threshold to neglect all clusters with the size smaller than 300 pixels. Therefore, in order to establish the presence of the lesions, the number of found components should be higher than 0, otherwise the image corresponds to a normal condition. Then, for localization of angiodysplasia lesions we return centroid coordinates of all connected components.

Table 15.1 Segmentation results. Intersection over Union (IoU) and Dice coefficient (Dice) are in %, and inference time (Time) is in ms

Model	IOU	Dice	Time
U-Net	73.18	83.06	30
TernausNet11	74.94	84.43	51
TernausNet16	73.83	83.05	60
AlbuNet34	**75.35**	**84.98**	**21**

15.4 Results

The qualitative results of segmentation and localization on the image from the validation set are shown in Fig. 15.2. Given imperfect segmentation, this example does show that the algorithm successfully detects angiodysplasia lesions. When there are few lesions in an image and they are well separated in space, the detector demonstrates near-perfect performance. In case of many lesions that possibly overlap in space, further improvements are required in order to achieve better performance, specifically in choosing model hyperparameters.

The quantitative comparison of our models' performance is presented in the Table 15.1. As measured by the segmentation performance, both modifications of TernausNet and AlbuNet34 demonstrate performance improvements over the original U-Net architecture. AlbuNet34 shows the overall best results with $IoU = 0.754$ and $Dice = 0.831$. These results show that despite the different image characteristics, networks pre-trained on natural images improve initialization of the encoder part in the segmentation model. When compared by the inference time, AlbuNet is also the fastest model due to the lighter encoder. This network takes around 20 ms to segment 512×512 pixel image and more than three times as fast as TernausNets. The inference time was measured using a single NVIDIA GTX 1080Ti GPU.

These results can be improved even further by, for example, employing deeper and/or wider encoder architectures (Iglovikov et al. 2018) and applying more sophisticated image augmentations.

The code of this methodology is publicly available under MIT license at https://github.com/ternaus/angiodysplasia-segmentation.

References

Chaurasia, A., & Culurciello, E. (2017). Linknet: Exploiting encoder representations for efficient semantic segmentation. arXiv preprint arXiv:1707.03718.

He, K., Zhang, X., Ren, S., & Sun, J. (2016). Deep residual learning for image recognition. In *Proceedings of the IEEE Conference on Computer Vision and Pattern Recognition* (pp. 770–778).

Iglovikov, V., & Shvets, A. (2018). TernausNet: U-net with VGG11 encoder pre-trained on imagenet for image segmentation. arXiv preprint arXiv:1801.05746.

Iglovikov, V. I., Rakhlin, A., Kalinin, A. A., & Shvets, A. A. (2018). Paediatric bone age assessment using deep convolutional neural networks. In *Deep Learning in Medical Image Analysis and Multimodal Learning for Clinical Decision Support* (pp. 300–308). Springer.

Iglovikov, V., Seferbekov, S., Buslaev, A., & Shvets, A. (2018, June). TernausNetV2: Fully convolutional network for instance segmentation. In *The IEEE Conference on Computer Vision and Pattern Recognition (CVPR) Workshops*.

Ronneberger, O., Fischer, P., & Brox, T. (2015). U-net: Convolutional networks for biomedical image segmentation. In *International Conference on Medical Image Computing and Computer-Assisted Intervention* (pp. 234–241). Springer.

Shvets, A. A., Rakhlin, A., Kalinin, A. A., & Iglovikov, V. I. (2018). Automatic instrument segmentation in robot-assisted surgery using deep learning. In *2018 17th IEEE International Conference on Machine Learning and Applications (ICMLA)*. IEEE.

Simonyan, K., & Zisserman, A. (2014). Very deep convolutional networks for large-scale image recognition. arXiv preprint arXiv:1409.1556.

Chapter 16
Regression-Based Convolutional Neural Network with a Tracker

Ruikai Zhang and Carmen C. Y. Poon

16.1 Motivation

An automatic colonic polyp localization algorithm named RYCO is developed to tackle the challenges of precise polyp location indication together with fast processing time when general limited and accessible computation resource is given. The uniqueness of RYCO is that it aims to utilize spatial information from current frame while incorporate temporal information accumulated from previous frames. Figure 16.1 shows the pipeline of RYCO, where a regression-based 2D CNN detection model named ResYOLO was built to locate a polyp in current frame as well as to check whether the tracked polyp was still in the view. Meanwhile, assuming that a polyp will not jump from one location to another between two consecutive frames by large distance, a DCF-based tracker called Efficient Convolution Operators (ECO) (Danelljan et al. 2017) was introduced to provide a stable guidance on the polyp location. The proposed pipeline is robust on frames with poor quality such as electrical noise and motion artifacts that are commonly encountered during colonoscopy. It has also inspired a few researchers adopting the same architecture with different CNN architectures and tracking methods for similar tasks.

R. Zhang (✉) · C. C. Y. Poon
Department of Surgery, The Chinese University of Hong Kong, Hong Kong, China
e-mail: rzhang@surgery.cuhk.edu.hk

J. Bernal and A. Histace (eds.), *Computer-Aided Analysis of Gastrointestinal Videos*,
https://doi.org/10.1007/978-3-030-64340-9_16

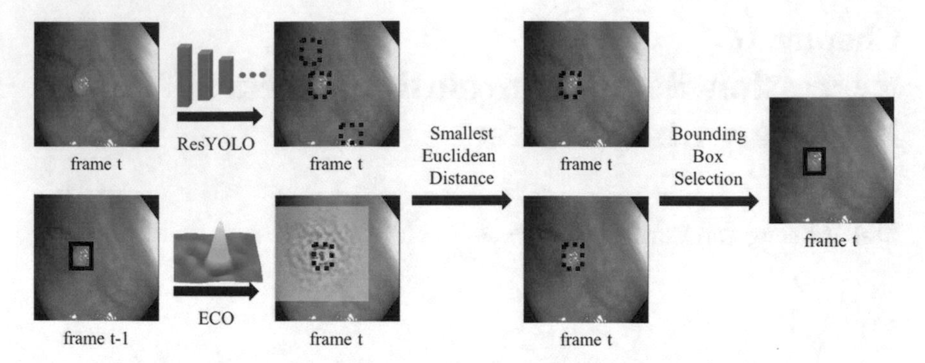

Fig. 16.1 Pipeline of the proposed computer-aided detection algorithm RYCO (Zhang et al. 2018)

16.2 Method Description in Details

16.2.1 Spatial Feature Learning

16.2.1.1 One-Stage Detector

It is reported that one-stage object detector can be at least 2.5 times faster than a region-proposal-based object detector with comparable performance (Redmon et al. 2016). In addition, regression-based CNN encodes information of the whole image instead of regions to make predictions and therefore, it is less vulnerable to background errors. The proposed regression-based 2D CNN ResYOLO is based on a famous one-stage object detector called YOLO (Redmon et al. 2016). Adopting the one-stage strategy, the intuition of YOLO was to mathematically model all ground truths in a single matrix, which make the end-to-end CNN training straightforward and efficient. Firstly, input image was divided into G by G grids, and the CNN model was trained to predict B bounding boxes for each grid. The ground truth for each grid to be assigned for training was decided by whether an object was centered on that grid. If the grid contained an object, the conditional class probability $P(c)$ for class c would be assigned. A total of five indicators were used to describe each bounding box, of which includes four indicators for box offset and one indicator for confidence score of objectness $Conf$. The box offset was described by object center coordinates (x, y), width, and height of the box (w, h). Thus, each grid was described by a vector of K elements, where $K = 5 \times B + C$. The output of candidate bounding boxes for the whole image was a matrix of size of $G \times G \times K$. Non-maximum suppression was used to remove redundant candidate bounding boxes with high intercept of union with each other. The loss function L for optimizing the regression model was comprised of loss for grids labeled as object L_{obj} and those as no-object L_{no-obj} described in the following equations:

$$L_{obj} = \sum_{g}^{G^2}(\sum_{b}^{B} O_{g,b}(\lambda_{bbox}\epsilon(x_g, y_g, \sqrt{w_g}, \sqrt{h_g}) + \epsilon(Conf_g)) + O_g \sum_{c}^{C} \epsilon(P_g(c))) \quad (16.1)$$

$$L_{no-obj} = \sum_{g}^{G^2}\sum_{b}^{B}(1 - O_{g,b})\lambda_{no-obj}(\epsilon(Conf_g)) \quad (16.2)$$

$$L = L_{obj} + L_{no-obj} \quad (16.3)$$

where g and b are the index for grid and box, respectively. The higher the intersection over union the predicted bounding box is with ground truth, the higher the $Conf$ is. Function $\epsilon(\cdot)$ denotes the sum of square of the differences between the variable and its ground truth. Indicator O equals to 1 if any object is within the selected grid and equals to 0 if not. As described above, since one-stage object detector trained regression on box offset and class probability as well as taking loss for grids with and without objects into account simultaneously, it is not fair to take the loss of different terms for equal contribution to the overall loss. Thus, different weights coefficient λ were added to different terms, where λ_{bbox} was associated to the loss for box offset and λ_{no-obj} was associated to loss of non-object. The different weights λ were selected according to (Redmon et al. 2016).

16.2.1.2 Residual Learning Module

Objects in non-medical domain usually stand out more clearly from the image background than objects in medical domain. In colonoscopic images, for example, a polyp usually looks very similar to its surrounding mucosa. In order to extract features that better describe endoscopic and histological features of different polyps, we proposed to introduce residual learning modules in the YOLO CNN architecture for feature learning (He et al. 2016). The rationale of including the residual learning modules in our design is as follows: It was reported that the depth of the CNN is crucial for performance as the more layers network has, the richer and more abstract the features can be learned, which could benefit in identifying polyps from mucosa. Nevertheless, as the CNN architecture gets deeper, it becomes more difficult to train, especially when only limited training data samples are available. By introducing the residual module as a skip network structure in the design, an enrich set of features can be extracted from the proposed deep architecture even with limited training data. The diagram of residual learning modules used in ResYOLO is illustrated in Fig. 16.2. The residual mapping $F(\cdot)$ implemented can be described by

$$H_l = F_l(H_{l-1}) + I(H_{l-1}) \quad (16.4)$$

where $I(\cdot)$ is the identity function, l is the index of layer, and H_l denotes the output of lth layer. Three convolutional blocks were used for residual feature learning, where a, b, c, and d were coefficients to manipulate the number of channels N and dimension S of the data. If both the number of channels and the dimensions of H_{l-1}

Fig. 16.2 Residual learning module of our proposed ResYOLO detector

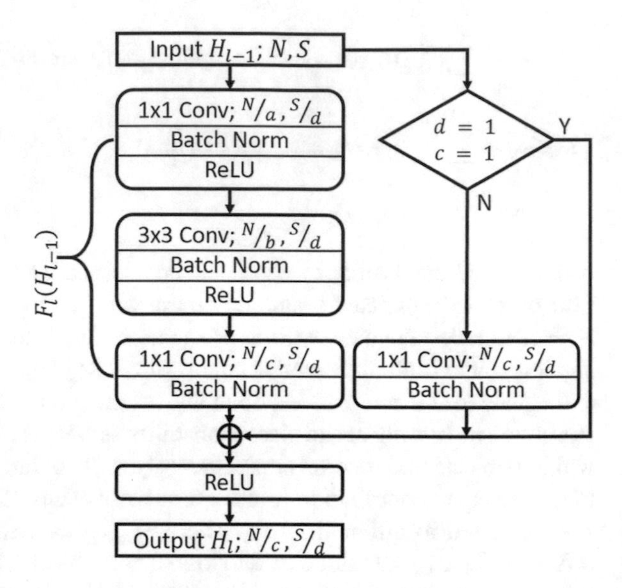

and H_l were the same, the identity function $I(\cdot)$ can be described as $I(x) = x$. While in some cases, coefficient c was set to 0.5 to increase the number of features to extract and d was set to 2 to down-sample instead of using pooling layers. To match up the size of $I(H_{l-1})$ with $F_l(H_{l-1})$, an additional 1×1 convolutional layer was added and the identity function $I(\cdot)$ was described as $I(x) = x$ instead.

16.2.1.3 Training of ResYOLO

The CNN-based object detectors were usually trained with images containing objects only in previous studies, while these detectors can still perform well as non-medical objects were usually visually special. However, polyps in endoscopic images can be wrongly identified or missed as they can sometimes be mixed up with normal mucosa or colon wall. It is intuitive to train the object detector with both endoscopic images with or without polyps, which introduce more variations to better extract features that are specific to polyps. Thus, besides images with polyps, images without polyps extracted from endoscopic videos were also included in the training dataset and labeled them as a negative class such that the number of classes C used in our model was 2 instead of 1, which is just the polyp. The benefits of including additional negative class are categorized in two folds: (1) the training dataset covers a more generalized data distribution; and (2) the trained model will be more sensitive to suspicious frames and reduce false positives.

Besides similarity of object to backgrounds, the quality of endoscopic video frames extracted also brings challenges to the training of ResYOLO. Although it's arguable whether polyps in images damaged by motion artefacts were worth detecting, regardless of the quality, all polyp images were accounted as long as the polyp can still be recognized in some degree in this training design. Besides using common augmentation methods for training dataset like random degree rotation, up-down flip, and left-right flip, two additional methods were used as well, which were additive Gaussian smoothing and random contrast and brightness for the purposed of mimicking the motion blurs caused by bowel and endoscope movements and variations of light conditions during colonoscopy. The sequence of methods used for augmentation was randomly selected during training. For example, some of the images were augmented by rotation of random degree, up-down flip, and Gaussian smoothing only, while some were augmented by all the five methods mentioned above. The degree of random rotation, Gaussian smoothing, and contrast and brightness were all randomly selected within a certain range to keep augmentation from going beyond reasons.

The diagram of architecture of ResYOLO detector was illustrated in Fig. 16.3, where 16 residual learning modules were used with three convolutional layers followed as classifier. The first and second numbers after each semicolon in each block of layers in Fig. 16.3 represents the number of channels and the dimension of the output, respectively. Images were resized to $448 \times 448 \times 3$ pixels and subtracted with the mean of training dataset as input. The grid size G is set to be 14, which was also the dimension of the output matrix. The intuition of using 14 instead of the original setting of using 7 in YOLO is to equip ResYOLO with a better capacity in identifying small polyps. Moreover, the number of candidate bounding boxes B predicted for each grid was set to 2 so that the number of channels of the output matrix was $12(5 * 2 + 2)$. The maximum number of objects can be detected in this configuration will be $392(14 * 14 * 2)$, which was considered more than enough and sufficient for polyp detection since the number of polyps appeared in the same endoscopic images rarely goes beyond 10.

16.2.2 Temporal Information Integration

16.2.2.1 Integration of ResYOLO Detector and ECO Tracker

To better explain how the results of ResYOLO detector and ECO tracker (Danelljan et al. 2017) were integrated, each frame was assumed to contain at most one polyp here. ECO tracker will only be activated once a polyp was detected by ResYOLO detector, of which the detection was confirmed by the candidate bounding box with the highest confidence score $Conf$ in the frame higher than a threshold T. Once the ECO tracker was activated, the final decision for a frame t was no longer decided by only ResYOLO detector but instead decided by two factors: (1) fusion of predictions resulted from both ResYOLO detector and ECO tracker, (2) predictions made from previous frames. The pipeline of this procedure can be summarized in Fig. 16.1. The candidate polyp location given by ECO tracker was used as a guidance for a rough location of polyp for frame t. To avoid miss detection on some polyp frames during a consecutive period, regardless of whether the $Conf$ score predicted was higher

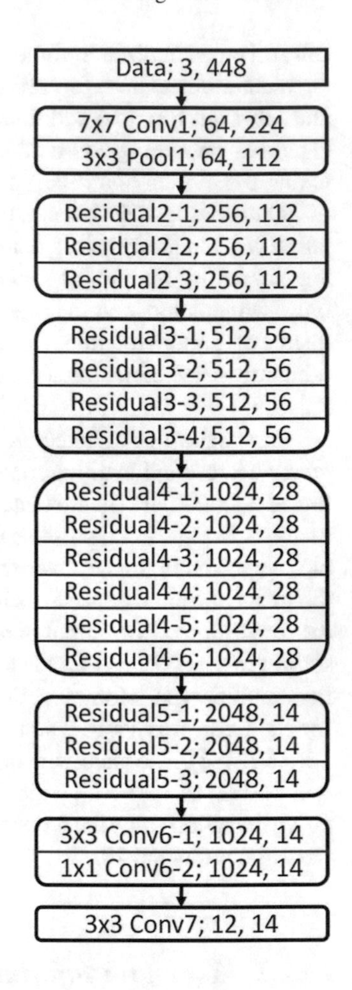

Fig. 16.3 Architecture of ResYOLO detector

than the threshold T or not, the one bounding box given by ResYOLO detector with the smallest Euclidean distance to the candidate polyp location given by ECO tracker was taken as a second candidate bounding box. If the mean $Conf$ of the previous M (including the one from current frame) frames that were predicted with polyps contained, denoted as $\overline{Conf}$, was larger than another threshold $\hat{T}$, then the current frame was suspicious of containing polyp; otherwise, stop ECO tracker and re-initialize it again when polyp was detected by ResYOLO on later frames. The intuition of using $\overline{Conf}$ is to refine the original $Conf$ of current prediction resulted from ResYOLO detector based on the temporal information brought by ECO tracker, where the additional threshold $\hat{T}$ for the refined $\overline{Conf}$ was using the same threshold T for $Conf$ for simplicity. The $\overline{Conf}$ is calculated by

$$\overline{Conf} = \frac{1}{M} * \sum_{m=0}^{M-1} Conf^{t-m} \tag{16.5}$$

If the $Conf^t$ of the selected candidate bounding box given by ResYOLO detector on current frame t was higher than the said $\overline{Conf}$, then this bounding box will be considered as the final detection for current frame t and used as one of the samples for online training of ECO tracker.

16.2.3 Experimental Setup

The models were trained using images with or without polyps to evaluate the performance improvement brought by introducing negative class. Similar to the optimizing strategy utilized in YOLO (Redmon et al. 2016), a smaller learning rate 10^{-5} was used for the first epoch, followed by a higher learning rate 10^{-4} and gradually decreased by a factor of 10. The decay rate, momentum, and batch size were set as 0.0005, 0.9 and 5, respectively. Threshold T for initializing tracking as well as determining suspicious frame was 0.2. The performance of using different numbers of frames M for calculating the $\overline{Conf}$ was reported. The best performance of RYCO resulted in M equals to 6.

References

Danelljan, M., Bhat, G., Khan, F. S., & Felsberg, M. (2014, July). ECO: Efficient convolution operators for tracking. In *2017 IEEE Conference on Computer Vision and Pattern Recognition (CVPR)* (pp. 417–422).

He, K., Zhang, X., Ren, S., & Sun, J. (2016). Deep residual learning for image recognition. In *Proceedings of the IEEE Conference on Computer Vision and Pattern Recognition* (pp. 770–778).

Redmon, J., Divvala, S., Girshick, R., & Farhadi, A. (2016, June). You only look once: Unified, real-time object detection. In *2016 IEEE Conference on Computer Vision and Pattern Recognition (CVPR)* (pp. 779–788).

Zhang, R., Zheng, Y., Poon, C., Shen, D., & Lau, J. (2018). Polyp detection during colonoscopy using a regression-based convolutional neural network with a tracker. *Pattern Recognition, 83*, 209–219.

Chapter 17
Other Methodologies

Jorge Bernal and Aymeric Histace

We present in this section some works belonging to teams that also took part in the different editions of GIANA challenge but, for time reasons, were not able to provide full chapters like the rest of teams.

17.1 GastroView Angiodysplasia Detection and Localization

Angiodysplasia detection algorithm in the GastroView system uses a convolutional neural network as a base classification model. The network is trained on image patches instead of entire images in order to operate in sliding-window mode in test time. The outputs are then aggregated and postprocessed in order to provide detection (full-frame classification) and localization outputs.

17.1.1 Base Model

Classification model uses MobileNet network architecture, featuring good tradeoff between accuracy and computational cost (Howard et al. 2017). In order to address

J. Bernal (✉)
Computer Vision Center and Computer Science Department, Universitat Autònoma de Barcelona, Bellaterra (Cerdanyola del Vallès), 08193 Barcelona, Spain
e-mail: Jorge.Bernal@uab.cat

A. Histace
ENSEA, ETIS UMR 8051, CY Paris Cergy University, CNRS,
6 av. du Ponceau, 95014 Cergy, France

J. Bernal and A. Histace (eds.), *Computer-Aided Analysis of Gastrointestinal Videos*,
https://doi.org/10.1007/978-3-030-64340-9_17

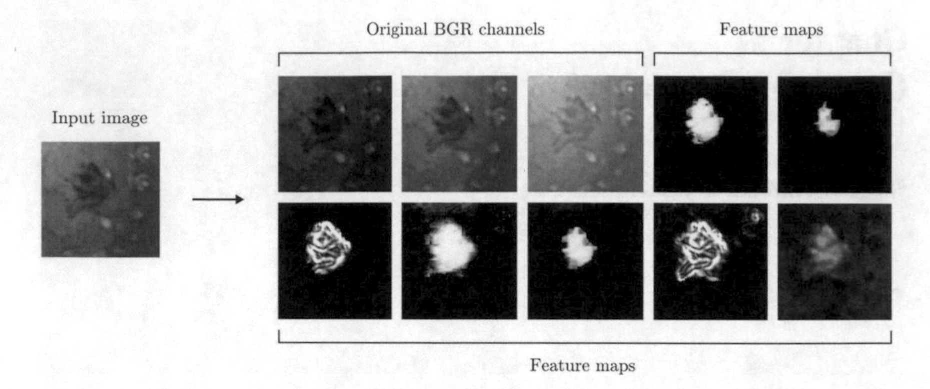

Fig. 17.1 Proposed feature maps for exemplary angiodysplasia image patch

the relatively low training data size, training of the base classification model is performed on image patches cropped from the original images, which significantly increases the amount of training samples (at the cost of losing some context information, however). Four rectangular patch sizes were used of following ratios: 0.1, 0,2, 0.33, 0.5. During training process, for each input image, several random patches are selected and put into the input batch. Also, batches are balanced in a positive-negative ratio of 1:2. In addition, input images are subject to random augmentation transforms, including rotation, flip, skew and perspective transforms, blur, noise as well as color variance transforms: hue distortion, saturation distortion, and PCA color augmentation (Krizhevsky et al. 2012).

As an additional mean for addressing low training data size, a concept of dedicated feature maps is introduced. For this purpose, seven high-level features of angiodysplasia were identified and implemented in a form of simple image processing algorithms. Each of the features produces an activation map. The resulting seven feature maps are appended to regular B, G, R channels of the original image, forming a 10-channel image, which is passed as input to the neural network, with feature maps suppressed with 0.1 factor in order to keep network focus on the original channels. The features are based on the previous work (Brzeski 2014) and they include three features detecting areas of high color similarity to angiodysplasia regions (based on smoothed histograms), including color similarity, area smoothness and contour clearness, similar set of three features for regions of moderate angiodysplasia color similarity, and lastly, a feature describing domination of red color. Figure 17.1 shows an example of the proposed feature maps applied over an input image.

After initial training of the classifier, hard example mining was applied, in which 30% of all training samples that produced worst classification results were selected and inserted into hard examples set. In the final training, training samples were picked in 1:1 ratio from the original training set and from the hard examples set, resulting in approximately four times amplification of hard examples in the training process. The final base classifier is an ensemble of six top performing models, each acquired from a different split of sixfold cross-validation applied over the training set.

17.1.2 *Detection*

In order to perform classification of a full image frame, a sliding-window detector using the base model is applied over the image, using patch sizes of 0.1, 0.2, 0.33, 0.5 and respective overlaps 0.5, 0.5, 0.5, 0.25. For each patch size a separate threshold value was defined. The final detector returns a positive output, if at least one base model output on any image patch exceeds the threshold respective for its size. The four thresholds were automatically optimized using random search to minimize full-frame classification error, evaluated using cross-validation over the training set.

17.1.3 *Localization*

The outputs of the base model collected over the image during the sliding-window process are converted into an activation map. To achieve this, each positive output from the detection is added to the activation map, while negative outputs are subtracted. In order to smooth the activation map, scores for patches are represented as circles instead of rectangles and blur is applied, which is followed by normalization of the map. The base model activation map is then multiplied by the fourth of the introduced feature maps, denoting moderate color values similarity to angiodysplasia regions, which results in the final activation map.

Next, for each patch size a new threshold value is defined. The final localization algorithm returns one angiodysplasia location point for each base model output that exceeds the threshold respective for its size, and the selected point is the location of maximum value of the activation map in the area of considered patch. Similarly as detection thresholds, localization thresholds are automatically optimized using cross-validation and random search to minimize localization error over the training set.

References

Brzeski, A. (2014). Visual features for endoscopic bleeding detection. *Current Journal of Applied Science and Technology*, 3902–3914.

Howard, A. G., Zhu, M., Chen, B., Kalenichenko, D., Wang, W., Weyand, T., Andreetto, M., & Adam, H. (2017). Mobilenets: Efficient convolutional neural networks for mobile vision applications. arXiv preprint arXiv:1704.04861.

Krizhevsky, A., Sutskever, I., & Hinton, G. E. (2012). ImageNet classification with deep convolutional neural networks. In F. Pereira, C. J. C. Burges, L. Bottou, & K. Q. Weinberger (Eds.), *Advances in neural information processing systems 25* (pp. 1097–1105). Curran Associates, Inc.

Part IV
Experimental Setup

Chapter 18
Polyp Detection in Colonoscopy Videos

Jorge Bernal, Gloria Fernández, Ana García-Rodríguez, Yael Tudela, Marina Riera, and F. Javier Sánchez

18.1 CVC-VideoClinicDB Dataset

We introduced in GIANA 2017 and 2018 challenges CVC-VideoClinicDB database, which is composed of 38 short and long sequences extracted from routinary explorations at Hospital Clinic of Barcelona, Spain using OLYMPUS endoscopes. This database aims to cover all different scenarios that a given support system should face. We provide an approximation of ground truth for all polyp frames, as shown in Fig. 18.2. Ground truth was created using GT Creator tool (Bernal et al. 2017).

CVC-ClinicVideoDB is the largest fully publicly available database[1] and contains a total of 29657 frames (21813 frames (73.55%) containing at least a polyp). Complete description of CVC-ClinicVideoDB is shown Fig. 18.1.

18.2 Performance Metrics

There are some terms defined next which are key to set performance metrics. As we deal with images from real patients examinations, we will find two different cases: images with polyps and images without polyps.

In the first case, if detection output lies within the polyp, the method is said to be providing a **True Positive (TP)** or correct alarm. It has to be noted that only one TP

[1] Available at https://giana.grand-challenge.org.

J. Bernal (✉) · Y. Tudela · M. Riera · F. J. Sánchez
Computer Vision Center and Computer Science Department, Universitat Autònoma de Barcelona, Bellaterra (Cerdanyola del Vallès), 08193 Barcelona, Spain
e-mail: Jorge.Bernal@uab.cat

G. Fernández · A. García-Rodríguez
Endoscopy Unit, Gastroenterology Department, ICMDiM, Hospital Clínic, IDIBAPS, CIBEREHD, University of Barcelona, Barcelona, Spain

J. Bernal and A. Histace (eds.), *Computer-Aided Analysis of Gastrointestinal Videos*,
https://doi.org/10.1007/978-3-030-64340-9_18

Training and Validation sets										Testing set									
ID	PF	NPF	PC	S	ID	PF	NPF	PC	S	ID	PF	NPF	PC	S	ID	PF	NPF	PC	S
1	386	112	0-Is	4	10	762	78	0-IIa	3	1	365	1351	0-Ip	9	10	191	0	0-Is	4
2	597	176	0-Is	6	11	370	130	0-Is	4	2	302	0	0-IIa	5	11	1185	0	0-Is	5
3	819	153	0-Is	8	12	261	124	0-IIa	3	3	638	52	0-Is	8	12	270	240	0-Is	9
4	350	40	0-Is	6	13	620	4	0-Is	4	4	921	99	0-IIa	4	13	327	0	0-Is	8
5	412	78	0-Is	5	14	2015	45	0-Is	6	5	1354	1256	0-Is	40	14	778	349	0-Ip	12
6	522	335	0-Ip	9	15	360	215	0-Is	6	6	454	0	0-Is	5	15	1103	71	0-Ip	10
7	738	103	0-Is	4	16	366	5	0-Is	3	7	1116	283	0-Ip	6	16	767	817	0-Is	3
8	405	44	0-IIa	5	17	651	146	0-IIa	5	8	773	187	0-IIa	8	17	1165	765	0-Ip	14
9	532	19	0-Ip	9	18	259	122	0-Ip	10	9	632	136	0-Is	9	18	251	535	0-Ip	10

Fig. 18.1 Statistics of CVC-ClinicVideoDB database. PF stands for polyp frames, NPF for non-polyp frames, PC for Paris classification representing morphology of the polyp according (0-Is for sessile polyps, 0-Ip for pedunculated polyps and 0-IIa for flat-elevated polyps) and S for the size of the polyps (in mm)

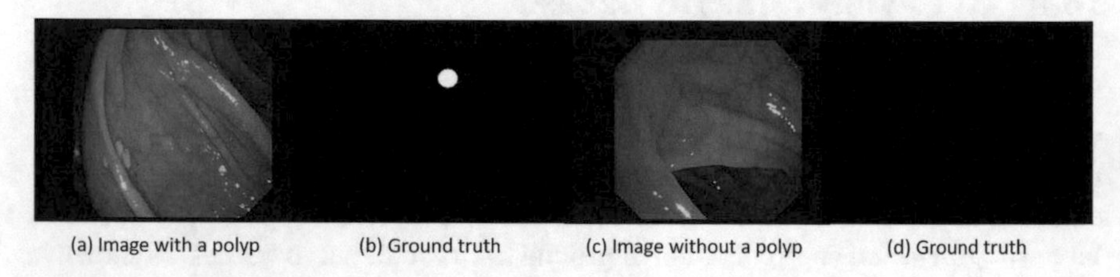

(a) Image with a polyp (b) Ground truth (c) Image without a polyp (d) Ground truth

Fig. 18.2 Example of the content of CVC-VideoClinicDB database. First pair of images shows a scene with a polyp and its corresponding binary ground truth mask, representing the polyp in the image. The second pair of images shows a scene without a polyp. In this case, ground truth is a black image

will be considered per polyp, no matter how many detections fall within the polyp. Any detection that falls outside the polyp is considered a **False Positive (FP)** or false alarm. The absence of alarm in images with a polyp is considered a **False Negative (FN)**, counting one per each polyp in the image that has not been detected. Regarding images without polyps, we define as a **True Negative (TN)** whenever the method does not provide any output for this particular image. Any detection provided for frames without a polyp counts as a **False Positive (FP)**. Considering these definitions, we propose the use of the frame-based performance metrics presented in Table 18.1.

Apart from these metrics, we will also use Reaction Time (RT) as a way to measure how fast a given system reacts to the presence of a polyp in the sequence. RT is calculated as the time difference (in frames) between the first appearance of the polyp in the sequence and the first correct detection/localization. Given that in results tables we will only show mean reaction time across all test sequences, we will calculate Mean Reaction Time (MRT) as the mean of all reaction times (not counting for the mean those videos in which the polyp was not detected).

Table 18.1 Performance metrics for polyp detection

Metric	Abbreviation	Calculation
Precision	Prec	$Prec = \frac{TP}{TP+FP}$
Recall	Rec	$Rec = \frac{TP}{TP+FN}$
Specificity	Spec	$Spec = \frac{TN}{FP+FN}$
Accuracy	Acc	$Acc = \frac{TP+TN}{TP+TN+FP+FN}$
F1-measure	F1	$F1 = \frac{2 \times Prec \times Rec}{Prec+Rec}$
F2-measure	F2	$F2 = \frac{5 \times Prec \times Rec}{4 \times Prec+Rec}$

Team	Polyp Detection	Polyp Localization
KM	✓	✓
LIP6	✓	✓
CUSURG	✓	✓
TA-MIT	✓	✓
NTNU	✓	✓
UCL	✓	✓

Fig. 18.3 List of participants in GIANA 2017 Challenge on the polyp detection and localization categories

18.3 Validation Experiments

In this context we will present both polyp detection and localization results. As mentioned before in this book, detection refers to the capability of a given system to determine object presence/absence in an image, without worrying about where the detected object is. Localization deals with the accurate identification of the area that occupies the polyp in the image.

18.4 Participating Teams

Figures 18.3 and 18.4 show the different teams that took part in the 2017 and 2018 iterations of the polyp detection and localization sub-challenges of GIANA. As it can be seen, 6 different teams took part in the first edition of this subchallenge, being this number increased to 14 in the 2018 edition.

Team	Polyp Detection	Polyp Localization
FanVoyage	✓	✓
KM	✓	✓
LIP6	✓	✓
LPixel	✓	✓
MIRC	✓	✓
MMMIL	✗	✓
ODS AI	✓	✓
OUS	✓	✓
PenguinAI	✓	✓
Rakhlin	✓	✓
RTC ATC	✓	✗
SRV UCL	✓	✓
Winterfell	✓	✓

Fig. 18.4 List of participants in GIANA 2018 Challenge on the polyp detection and localization categories

Reference

Bernal, J., Histace, A., Masana, M., Angermann, Q., Sánchez-Montes, C., de Miguel, C. R., et al. (2019). Gtcreator: A flexible annotation tool for image-based datasets. *International Journal of Computer Assisted Radiology and Surgery*, *14*(2), 191–201.

Chapter 19
Polyp Segmentation in Colonoscopy Images

Jorge Bernal, Gloria Fernández, Ana García-Rodríguez, and F. Javier Sánchez

19.1 CVC-HDSegment, CVC-300 Y CVC-612 Datasets

With respect to polyp segmentation, two different types of data will be provided: Standard-Definition (SD, $574 \times 500 \times 3$ and $384 \times 288 \times 3$ pixels) images and High-Definition (HD, $1920 \times 1080 \times 3$ pixels) images. We provide both of them to cover those cases that a given system might face during the exploration. Giving a first indication of the polyp region during the exploration might need to be under real-time constraints whether, once the polyp is found, the segmentation might be refined using HD images.

With respect to SD images, we propose the use of CVC-ColonDB (Bernal et al. 2012) as training dataset and CVC-ClinicDB (Bernal et al. 2015) as testing dataset. The training dataset contains 300 images all of them containing a polyp whereas the testing one contains 612 images that contain at least a polyp. We show examples of the content of both databases in Fig. 19.1.

We introduced in GIANA 2017 Sub-challenge the new CVC-PolypHD database,[1] which is the first, up to our knowledge, database for polyp segmentation comprising exclusively HD images. This database is composed of around 164 HD frames, 56 in the training set and 108 in the testing set, all of them showing a different polyp extracted from routinary explorations at Hospital Clinic of Barcelona, Spain. This database aims to cover as many different polyp appearances as possible. As ground truth, we provide a pixel-wise representation of the polyp region for all frames; this

[1] Available at https://giana.grand-challenge.org.

J. Bernal (✉) · F. J. Sánchez
Computer Vision Center and Computer Science Department, Universitat Autònoma de Barcelona, Bellaterra (Cerdanyola del Vallès), 08193 Barcelona, Spain
e-mail: Jorge.Bernal@uab.cat

G. Fernández · A. García-Rodríguez
Endoscopy Unit, Gastroenterology Department, ICMDiM, Hospital Clínic, University of Barcelona, IDIBAPS, CIBEREHD, Barcelona, Spain

J. Bernal and A. Histace (eds.), *Computer-Aided Analysis of Gastrointestinal Videos*,
https://doi.org/10.1007/978-3-030-64340-9_19

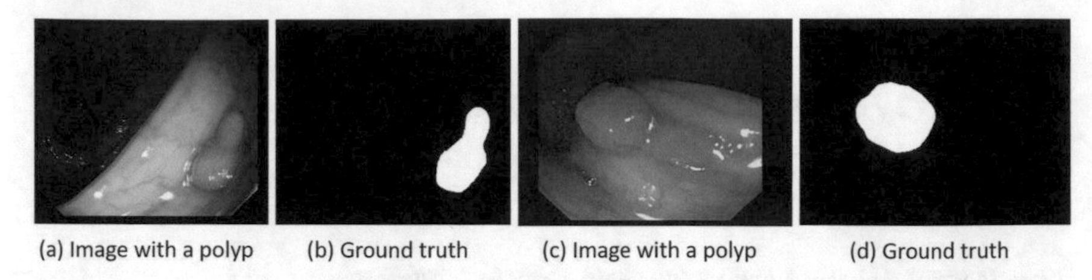

(a) Image with a polyp (b) Ground truth (c) Image with a polyp (d) Ground truth

Fig. 19.1 Examples of content of SD segmentation training and testing datasets. The first two images show an original image and its corresponding ground truth from CVC-ColonDB whereas the last two ones show an original image from CVC-ClinicDB and its corresponding ground truth

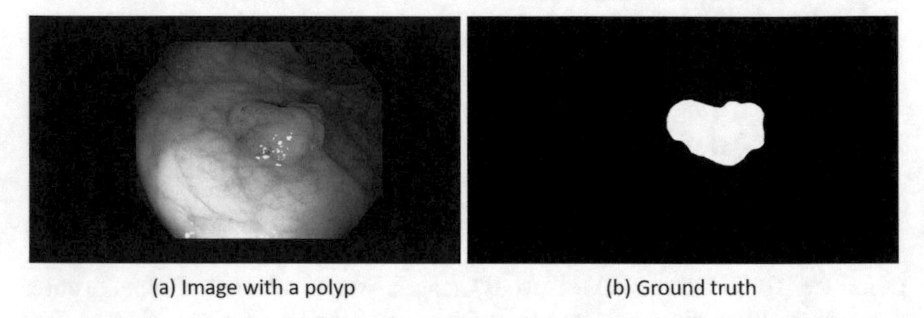

(a) Image with a polyp (b) Ground truth

Fig. 19.2 Examples of content of HD segmentation image dataset. Image on the left shows an original image showing a polyp whereas image on the right shows its associated binary mask annotation

ground truth was created using GT Creator software (Bernal et al. 2019). We show an example of the content of this database in Fig. 19.2.

19.2 Performance Metrics

With respect to the evaluation of polyp segmentation methods, we propose the use of state-of-the-art performance metrics: Jaccard and DICE similarity score. Jaccard index (also known as intersection over union, IoU) is defined as the size of the intersection divided by the size of the union of the sample sets, and it is calculated as follows:

$$J(method, gt) = \frac{|method \bigcap gt|}{|method \bigcup gt|}, \quad (19.1)$$

where method stands for the binary mask representing the output provided by the method and gt stands for the binary mask provided by clinicians as the ground truth annotation of the polyp region.

DICE similarity score is a statistic also used for comparing the similarity of two samples. It is calculated as follows:

Team	Polyp Detection	Polyp Localization
TA-MIT	✓	✓
NII	✓	✗
SFU	✓	✓
UCL	✓	✓
CVML	✓	✓

Fig. 19.3 List of participants in GIANA 2017 Challenge on polyp segmentation (SD and HD categories)

$$DICE(method, gt) = \frac{2|method \bigcap gt|}{|method| + |gt|}. \quad (19.2)$$

We propose the use of both scores as they consider in a different way the number of true positive pixels (those which coincide in the output and in the ground truth). DICE is also used to specify the amount of relevant information that is kept, which is crucial for the segmentation task as we mentioned before.

19.3 Validation Experiments

The experiments related to polyp segmentation aim to validate method performance in standard- and high-definition datasets. For each team we provide both mean and standard deviation values of the two considered performance metrics.

19.4 Participating Teams

Figures 19.3 and 19.4 show the different teams that took part in the 2017 and 2018 iterations of the polyp detection and localization sub-challenges of GIANA. As it happened for the polyp detection and localization sub-challenges, the number of participating teams grows from one edition to another, counting with 5 teams in the first one and 13 in the second one.

Team	Segmentation SD	Segmentation HD
CVML	✓	✓
FanVoyage	✓	✓
KM	✓	✓
MIRC	✓	✓
Modulabs	✓	✗
ODS AI	✓	✓
OUS	✓	✓
PenguinAI	✓	✓
Rakhlin	✓	✓
Reutlingen	✓	✗
SRV UCL	✓	✓
Winterfell	✓	✓
XMU-Insight	✗	✓

Fig. 19.4 List of participants in GIANA 2018 Challenge on polyp segmentation (SD and HD categories)

References

Bernal, J., Sánchez, J., & Vilarino, F. (2012). Towards automatic polyp detection with a polyp appearance model. *Pattern Recognition*, *45*(9), 3166–3182.

Bernal, J., Sánchez, F. J., Fernández-Esparrach, G., Gil, D., Rodríguez, C., & Vilariño, F. (2015). Wm-dova maps for accurate polyp highlighting in colonoscopy: Validation vs. saliency maps from physicians. *Computerized Medical Imaging and Graphics*, *43*, 99–111.

Bernal, J., Histace, A., Masana, M., Angermann, Q., Sánchez-Montes, C., de Miguel, C. R., et al. (2019). Gtcreator: A flexible annotation tool for image-based datasets. *International Journal of Computer Assisted Radiology and Surgery*, *14*(2), 191–201.

Chapter 20
Wireless Capsule Endoscopy Image Analysis

Aymeric Histace, Romain Leenhardt, and Xavier Dray

20.1 CAD-CAP Database

The Computer-Assisted Diagnosis for Capsule Endoscopy Database (CAD-CAP) is a French national multicenter database approved by the French Data Protection Authority in which still frames (associated with short adjacent video sequences) collected from 4,166 deidentified, third-generation SB-VCE videos (PillcamÂ® SB3 system, Medtronic) routinely recorded in 13 French centers can be found. This database comprises 6,360 still frames with a pathological finding (from 1,341 SB-VCEs).

In September 2016, all third-generation SB-CE videos (PillcamÂ® SB3 system, Medtronic, MN) registered in the 12 participating endoscopy units were retrospectively collected and deidentified. Clinical data were noted (age, gender, indication for SB-CE). Any SB icon selected by the local reared was considered as a frame of interest. Each frame of interest was extracted and included in the CAD-CAP database, together with a short adjacent video sequence that included 25 frames upstream and downstream the index frame. Two pre-med students were trained, and supervised by an expert reader, to select and to delimitate any lesion found into the selected frames of interest. The delimitation process used Adobe Photoshop CS6Â® (Adobe Systems, USA) and GIMPÂ® softwares (GNOME Foundation, USA) with a WacomÂ® (Wacom Co., Ltd, Japan) pen tablet connected to a laptop. During several face-to-face meetings, three expert SB-CE readers screened all selected frames of interest (and associated short video sequences) and all delimitations of abnormal findings within each selected frames. Doubtful, blurred, or irrelevant frames were

A. Histace (✉)
ENSEA, ETIS UMR 8051 (CY Paris Cergy University, ENSEA, CNRS),
6 av. du Ponceau, 95014 Cergy, France
e-mail: aymeric.histace@ensea.fr

R. Leenhardt · X. Dray
Hôpital Saint Antoine (APHP), Paris Sorbonne Université, ETIS UMR 8051 (CY Paris Cergy University, ENSEA, CNRS), 6 av. du Ponceau, 95014 Cergy, France

J. Bernal and A. Histace (eds.), *Computer-Aided Analysis of Gastrointestinal Videos*,
https://doi.org/10.1007/978-3-030-64340-9_20

excluded. Findings' delimitations were also reviewed, and remade when necessary. Abnormal findings were first sorted into three different categories: (a) fresh blood and clots; (b) vascular findings; and (c) ulcerative/inflammatory findings. Then, into these categories, all abnormal findings were sorted again according to their relevance. Relevance was defined as followed by a group of four SB-CE experts. Fresh blood and clots, typical angiectasia, and ulcerated lesions were considered "highly relevant" findings. Non-ulcerated but inflammatory findings (for instance, erythema, edema, denudation) were considered "moderately relevant" findings. Subtle vascular lesions (for instance, erythematous patches, red spots/dots, phlebectasia, and so-called "diminutive angiectasia") were considered "poorly relevant" findings.

A set of 20 normal and complete SB-CE videos was used to create a control dataset. Still frames were automatically extracted from these latter videos, every 1% of the SB sequence (between 1% and 100% of the SB sequence). Thus, 100 normal frames were extracted per video. Again, for any normal extracted still frame, a short video sequence was also captured (with 25 frames upstream and downstream the index frame). All supposedly normal frames were reviewed by two readers. Doubtful, blurred, or irrelevant frames were excluded.

We collected 4,174 third-generation SB-CE from the 12 participating centers. We included in the database 1,480 videos (35%) containing at least one frame of interest (with abnormal findings), and 20 normal videos (as controls). Clinical characteristics from these 1480 SB-CE were collected (59% men, 41% female, mean age of 64-year-old). SB-CE were mainly indicated for obscure gastrointestinal bleeding (67%), suspected Crohnâ's disease (CD) (12%), and sometimes (21%) for others various indications such as coeliac disease and Peutz–Jeghers polyposis. In total, we extracted 6,013 still frames (with their adjacent short video sequences). Abnormal findings were delimitated by the pre-med students within 5,124 frames, and then reviewed and sorted by the experts: 3103 frames contained images of vascular abnormalities (817 frames with highly relevant images of angiectasia, 2286 frames with other, poorly relevant, images of vascular lesions), 1370 frames contained images of ulcerative/inflammatory findings (1057 frames with highly relevant images of ulcerated lesions, 313 frames with moderately relevant images of inflammatory but not ulcerated lesions). Seven-hundred-and-eighteen frames contained highly relevant images of fresh blood and clots.

In the context of GIANA 2017, a first extraction was made from the CAD-CAP database to propose the following training and testing datasets focusing on angiectasia detection and localization:

- *Training2017*: 300 images presenting with typical angiectasia and 300 normal images;
- *Testing2017*: Same proportion as Training.

In the context of GIANA 2018, to make the tasks more challenging and in accordance with the clinical expectations, we proposed a third class to be considered focusing on inflammatory lesions. The database was composed in total of 1800 images that were divided into a training and a testing dataset as follows:

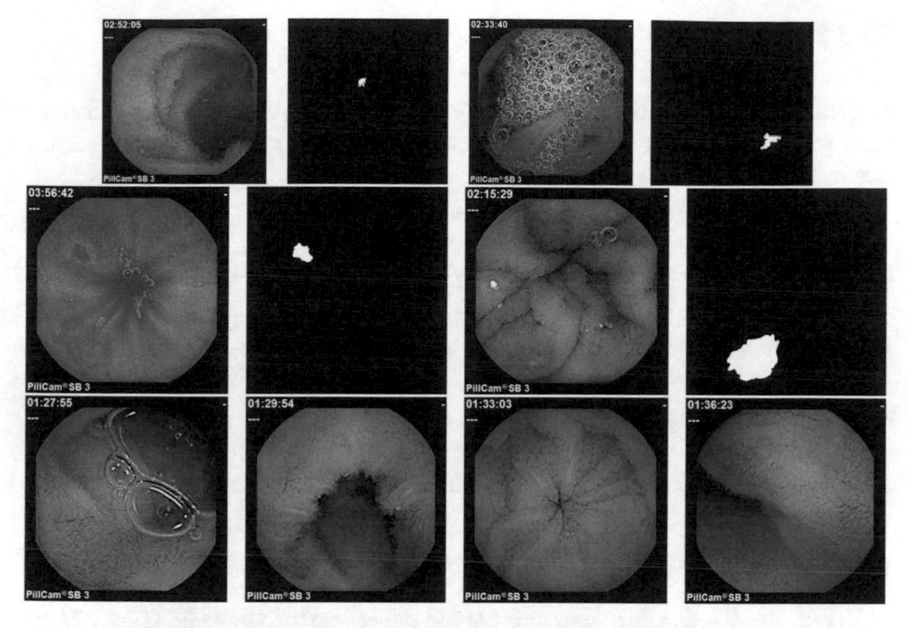

Fig. 20.1 Some examples of WCE images extracted from the CAD-CAP database with related ground truth. First raw: Angiectasia, Second raw: Inflammatory lesions, Third raw: Normal images

- *Training2018*: 300 images presenting with typical angiectasia, 300 presenting with typical inflammatory lesions (including ulcers), and 300 normal images;
- *Testing2018*: Same proportion as Training.

Some examples for each class are shown in Fig. 20.1.

20.2 Performance Metrics

20.2.1 GIANA 2017

As the proposed tasks for GIANA 2017 were related only on one specific lesion, the classic metrics were used for each tasks, that is to say:

- Precision, Recall, Specificity, Accuracy;
- F1, F2 scores;
- Area Under the ROC Curve (AUC) if a confidence value was provided by competitors.

20.2.2 GIANA 2018

In 2018, as the tasks evolved with integration of a new class, considering the detection task, the confusion matrix was used to provide more adapted metrics. The classic confusion matrix is shown in Fig. 20.2.

The following related metrics were used:

- Global Accuracy $= 100 \times \frac{A+E+I}{A+B+C+D+E+F+G+H+I}$,
- Normal Image Accuracy (NAI) $= 100 \times \frac{A+E+I}{A+B+C+D+E+G+I}$,
- Inflammatory Images Accuracy (IIA) $= \frac{A+E+I}{E+A+I+H+D+F}$,
- Vascular Images Accuracy (VIA) $= \frac{A+E+I}{I+E+A+C+F+G+H}$,
- Mean Accuracy per Class $= \frac{NIA+IIA+VIA}{3}$.

For the localization task, we came back to a more classic evaluation (see GIANA 2017) considering each class versus the rest of the images.

		Method Output		
		Normal	Inflammatory	Vascular
Ground Truth	Normal	A	B	C
	Inflammatory	D	E	F
	Vascular	G	H	I

Fig. 20.2 Confusion Matrix for GIANA 2018

Table 20.1 2017 Participating Team

Team	WCE Lesion Detection	WCE Lesion Localization
TA-MIT	✓	✓
KM	✓	✓
PG	✓	✓
NTNU	✓	✓
UCL	✓	✓
TUe	✓	✓
UMinho	✓	✓

Table 20.2 2018 Participating Team

Team	WCE Lesion Detection	WCE Lesion Localization
FanVoyage	✓	✓
KM	✓	✓
ODS_AI	✓	✓
PenguinAI	✓	✓
SRV UCL	✓	✓
TU/e-VCA	✓	✗
UB	✓	✗
Yimei	✗	✓

20.3 Participating Teams

In 2017, seven teams took part in the two tasks of the WCE challenge (see Table 20.1).

In 2017, eight teams took part in the WCE challenge (see Table 20.2), and five considered both detection and localization tasks. Three of them only took part to one task.

Part V
Experimental Results and Analysis

Chapter 21
Polyp Detection in Colonoscopy Videos

Jorge Bernal, Yael Tudela, Marina Riera, and F. Javier Sánchez

21.1 Polyp Detection and Localization

We present in this section results of the polyp detection and localization subchallenges, part of GIANA challenge. We will first make a separate analysis of the results per edition and last, we will show a summary of the main findings after analyzing the performances of the different teams. It has to be noted that some of the teams took part in different editions of the challenge under different names; in this case, we will use the best results of the team in the final summary.

21.1.1 GIANA 2017 Challenge

We can extract the following conclusions after analyzing Table 21.1. The main result that can be extracted is that all teams detect all polyps in at least one frame so no object is fully misdetected.

Going into details for each of the teams we can observe that LIP6 team is the one that detects more polyp frames but, when it comes to polyp localization, fails to place correctly the output inside the polyp. As a general trend, we can observe a decrease in all metrics when going from detection to localization task though it has to be mentioned that this seems to affect more KM and LIP6 teams than the rest.

The number of false alarms (and, therefore, precision score) is crucial for a potential deployment of these systems in the exploration room; in this context, TA-MIT, UCL, and CUSURG offer precision scores higher than 90%; these results do get worse for the localization sub-task where all teams see how their precision score is lowered by at least a 10%.

J. Bernal (✉) · Y. Tudela · M. Riera · F. J. Sánchez
Computer Vision Center and Computer Science Department, Universitat Autònoma de Barcelona, Bellaterra (Cerdanyola del Vallès), 08193 Barcelona, Spain
e-mail: Jorge.Bernal@uab.cat

J. Bernal and A. Histace (eds.), *Computer-Aided Analysis of Gastrointestinal Videos*,
https://doi.org/10.1007/978-3-030-64340-9_21

Table 21.1 Polyp detection and localization results at GIANA 2017. Total number of images: 18103 (12592 with a polyp and 6141 without a polyp)

Team	TP	FP	TN	FN	Prec	Rec	Spec	Acc	F1	F2	MRT
Polyp detection											
KM	8926	1545	4596	3666	85.2	70.9	74.8	72.2	77.4	73.3	3.72
ODS_AI - MIT	9471	862	5279	3121	91.7	75.2	85.9	78.7	82.6	78.0	14.0
LIP6	**11240**	3762	2379	**1352**	74.9	**89.2**	38.7	72.7	81.5	**85.9**	3.7
NTNU	10058	1282	4859	2534	88.7	79.8	79.1	**79.6**	**84.0**	81.5	**2.0**
UCL	9251	**766**	**5375**	3341	**92.3**	73.4	**87.5**	78.0	81.8	76.6	12.6
CUENDO	8812	928	5213	3780	90.5	69.9	84.9	74.9	78.9	73.3	10.3
Polyp localization											
KM	6267	4204	4596	6413	59.8	49.4	52.2	50.5	54.1	51.2	13.0
ODS_AI - MIT	8657	**1676**	5279	4023	**83.7**	68.2	75.9	**70.9**	75.2	70.9	37.3
LIP6	3650	11355	2375	9030	24.3	28.8	17.3	22.8	26.4	27.7	73.3
NTNU	**9287**	2053	4859	**3393**	81.9	**73.2**	70.3	72.2	**77.3**	**74.8**	**3.8**
UCL	8502	2226	**5375**	4178	79.2	67.0	70.7	68.4	72.6	69.2	13.4
CUENDO	8080	1660	5213	4600	82.9	63.7	**75.8**	67.9	72.1	66.8	13.0

With respect to aggregation metrics in polyp detection, we can observe how two teams provide superior performance than the rest by obtaining F1 and F2 scores higher than 80%. It is curious to see that, for polyp detection, LIP6 is the one achieving higher F2 score but NTNU outperforms them in the F1 score, though the difference is not big. For sure these results decrease when localization task is considered; in this case, NTNU appears as the best performing team obtaining both the highest F1 and F2 scores.

Finally, the analysis of MRT yields some interesting conclusions; in general, none of the teams take more than 1 second (25 frames) to alert polyp presence in the image, which could be seen as an almost instantaneous response to the stimuli. This good result is kept for the majority of teams when it comes to polyp localization; it is interesting to observe how UCL team almost keeps intact its MRT score, being NTNU the fastest team when alerting correctly of both polyp presence and location within the image.

These results are confirmed by the analysis of the ROC curves presented in Fig. 21.1. With respect to the lines representing each of the teams it has to be noted that some teams did not provide confidence values for their detections, being their performance represented by a single point. We can observe again the superior performance by LIP6 and NTNU for polyp detection and NTNU and TA-MIT for polyp localization.

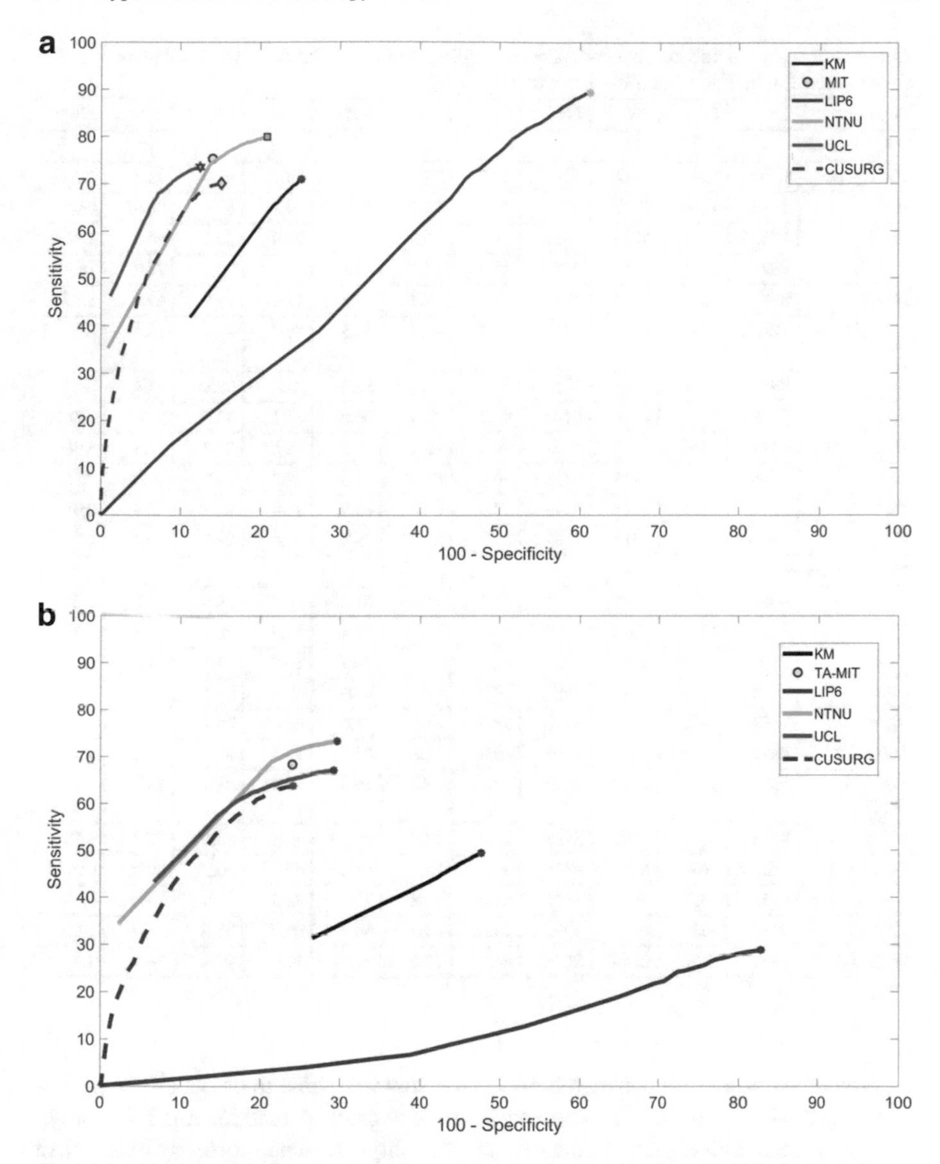

Fig. 21.1 ROC curves for **a** polyp detection and **b** polyp localization from GIANA 2017 challenge

21.1.2 GIANA 2018 Challenge

The year that passed between the two iterations of GIANA challenge leads to an increase in the number of participating teams and also in the performances achieved by the different methodologies presented. As we did for the previous edition, we highlight next the main conclusions that can be extracted (Table 21.2).

Table 21.2 Polyp detection and localization results at GIANA 2018. Total number of images: 18103 (12592 with a polyp and 6141 without a polyp)

Team	TP	FP	TN	FN	Prec	Rec	Spec	Acc	F1	F2	MRT
Polyp detection											
FanVoyage	9495	799	5342	3097	92.2	75.4	86.9	79.2	82.9	78.3	5.06
KM	**12193**	4440	1701	**399**	73.3	**96.8**	27.7	74.2	83.4	**90.9**	**0.06**
LIP6	11059	3923	2218	1533	73.8	87.8	36.1	70.9	80.2	84.6	3.83
LPixel	8822	1097	5044	3770	88.9	70.1	82.1	74.0	78.4	73.2	18.72
MIRC	8277	934	5207	4315	89.9	65.7	84.8	71.2	75.9	69.5	8.72
ODS_AI-MIT	10152	829	5312	2440	92.4	80.6	86.5	**82.5**	**86.1**	82.7	7.22
NTNU	9963	860	5281	2629	92.0	79.1	86.0	81.4	85.1	81.4	6.22
TencentAI	3448	**11**	**6130**	9144	**99.7**	27.4	**99.8**	51.1	42.9	32.0	259.19
Neuromation	9471	1416	4725	3121	86.9	75.2	76.9	75.8	80.7	77.3	5.06
RTC ATC	10174	3206	2935	2418	76.0	80.8	47.8	69.9	78.3	79.8	0.56
SRV UCL	10449	2094	4047	2143	83.3	82.9	65.9	77.4	83.1	83.0	0.61
Winterfell	11060	2531	3610	1532	81.4	87.8	58.8	78.3	84.5	86.4	1.22
Polyp localization											
FanVoyage	9056	1238	5342	3624	87.9	71.4	81.2	74.7	78.8	74.2	5.28
KM	9496	4055	3662	3184	70.0	74.9	47.4	64.5	72.4	73.8	4.11
LIP6	2403	12579	2218	10277	16.0	18.9	14.9	16.8	17.3	18.3	191.65
LPixel	7794	2644	5044	4886	74.7	61.4	65.6	63.0	67.4	63.7	35.22
MIRC	7782	2132	5298	4898	78.5	61.3	71.3	65.0	68.9	64.2	9.78
MMMIL	**9875**	1630	5078	**2805**	85.8	**77.8**	75.7	77.1	**81.6**	**79.3**	4.17
ODS_AI-MIT	9637	1344	5312	3043	87.7	76.0	79.8	**77.3**	81.4	78.1	18.89
NTNU	9478	1345	5281	3202	87.6	74.7	79.7	76.4	80.6	77.0	6.39
TencentAI	3255	**204**	**6130**	9425	**94.1**	25.6	**96.8**	49.3	40.3	30.0	256.87
Neuromation	9355	1959	4813	3325	82.7	73.8	71.0	72.8	77.9	75.4	9.78
SRV UCL	9288	3255	4047	3392	74.0	73.2	55.4	66.7	73.6	73.4	2.00
Winterfell	9842	5450	2564	2838	64.3	77.6	31.9	59.9	70.4	74.5	**1.78**

First of all, and as it happened before, all teams were able to detect all the polyps that appeared throughout the sequences. With respect to reaction time for polyp detection, almost all teams are able to detect the polyp presence correctly in less than a second (KM takes 0.06 frames only to detect the polyp); we can observe how one team (PenguinAI) has a way superior MRT than the rest of the teams. This happens because, in one sequence, the polyp appears and disappears and this particular team was only able to detect polyp apparition in the second sub-sequence.

With respect to correct detections we can observe how KM team is able to detect almost all polyp frames, followed by LIP6 which also offered a good performance in these terms in 2017. Again, the number of correct detections drops when we also consider good localizations; in this case, ODS_AI is the one that sees the smallest impact in performance when switching between both tasks.

Precision scores are clearly higher for polyp detection than for polyp localization, increasing vastly the number of false alarms when polyp localization is considered but for KM team, which is able to reduce the number of false alarms by increasing greatly the number of TN.

Finally, aggregation metrics are the ones that help us to determine which of the teams provided better overall performance. In this context, we can observe how KM is the one with better trade-off for polyp detection between F1 and F2 scores (specially due to its very high F2 score) whereas MMMIL is the one providing superior performance for the polyp localization task.

In order to confirm these results in a graphical way, we show in Fig. 21.2 ROC curves for polyp detection and localization associated to the results of GIANA 2018 challenge. We can clearly observe how KM distances from the rest of the teams with respect to polyp detection and how MMMIL outperforms the rest of the teams (being followed closely by $ODS\%_A I$) for the case of polyp localization.

21.2 Evolution of Results

Table 21.3 shows a summary of the most relevant findings after two iterations of the polyp detection sub-task as part of the GIANA challenge. First, we can observe that the performance of the best team (which were LIP6 in 2017 and KM in 2018) improves over the years. KM outperforms LIP6 in the most clinically relevant metrics (Recall, F1 and F2 scores, and MRT) though it has to be noted that it provides a higher number of false positives than LIP6.

This table also shows the evolution in the performance for those teams that concurred in both editions of GIANA. We can observe that, in general, they improved their performance, which can be particularly seen in the evolution of F1 and F2 scores. We want to emphasize that some teams improved their performance regarding MRT score by a great margin (KM, ODS_AI and, especially, UCL) which indicates that efforts were made to capture those more difficult polyp appearances which tend to happen when they first appear on screen.

We perform a similar analysis for the polyp localization task by observing carefully Table 21.3. Again we observe that the performance achieved by the best team (MMMIL in 2018 with respect to NTNU in 2017) improves year over year in all metrics but, surprisingly, on MRT. In this case, all performance metrics increase by a margin of around 4%, reducing the number of false alarms while detecting correctly more polyps.

With respect to the evolution per team, we observe how KM was able to greatly increase its polyp localization performance, increasing precision and recall metrics in more than 10 points. The rest of the teams also improved their performance with respect to the previous edition, particularly with respect of MRT and TP, leading to a consequent improvement in Recall, F1 and F2 scores (Table 21.4).

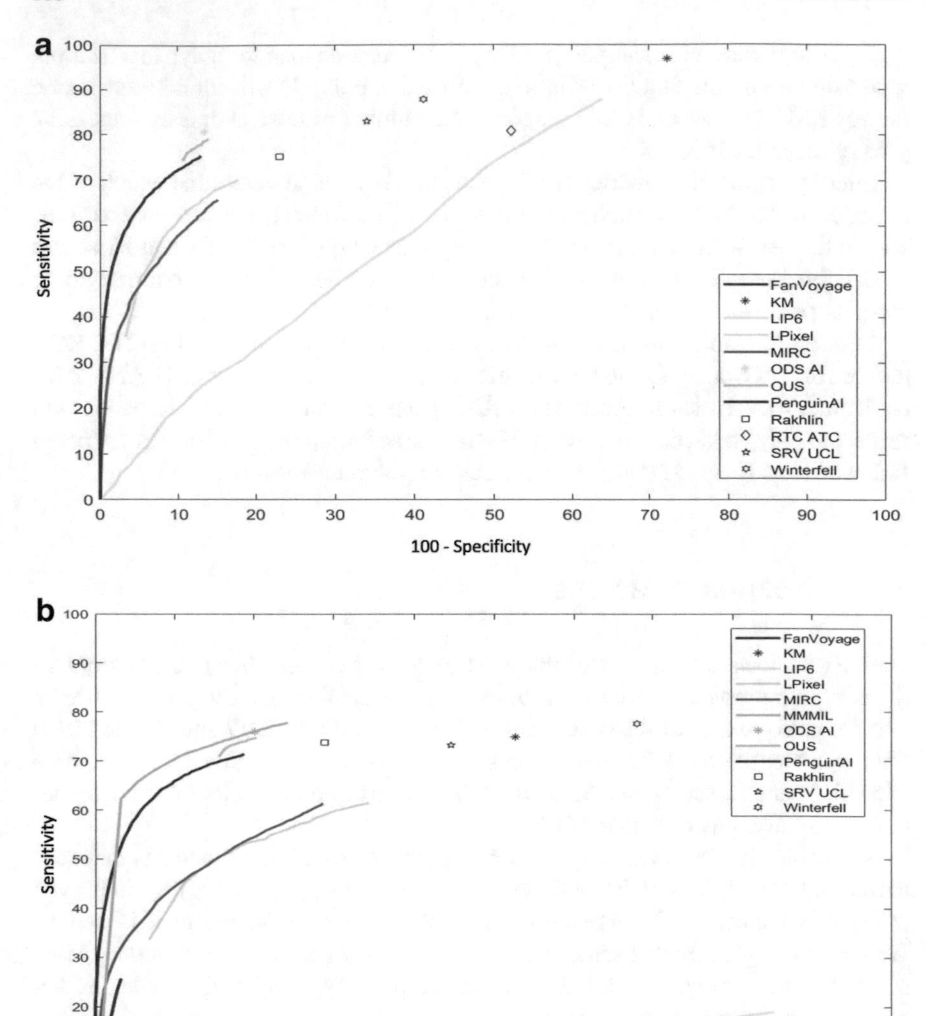

Fig. 21.2 ROC curves for **a** polyp detection and **b** polyp localization from GIANA 2018 challenge

Table 21.3 Summary of key results from the polyp detection task at GIANA 17 and 18 challenges

Year	Team	TP	FP	TN	FN	Prec	Rec	Spec	Acc	F1	F2	MRT
Best teams												
2017	LIP6	11240	**3762**	**2379**	1352	**74.9**	89.2	**38.7**	72.7	81.5	85.9	3.7
2018	KM	**12193**	4440	1701	**399**	73.3	**96.8**	27.7	**74.2**	**83.4**	**90.9**	**0.06**
Performance evolution												
2017	KM	8926	1545	4596	3666	85.2	70.9	74.8	72.2	77.4	73.3	3.72
2018	KM	12193	4440	1701	399	73.3	96.8	27.7	74.2	83.4	90.9	0.06
2017	ODS_AI - MIT	9471	862	5279	3121	91.7	75.2	85.9	78.7	82.6	78.0	14.0
2018	$ODS\_AI - MIT$	10152	829	5312	2440	92.4	80.6	86.5	82.5	86.1	82.7	7.22
2017	LIP6	11240	3762	2379	1352	74.9	89.2	38.7	72.7	81.5	85.9	3.7
2018	LIP6	11059	3923	2218	1533	73.8	87.8	36.1	70.9	80.2	84.6	3.83
2017	NTNU	10058	1282	4859	2534	88.7	79.8	79.1	79.6	84.0	81.5	2.0
2018	NTNU	9963	860	5281	2629	92.0	79.1	86.0	81.4	85.1	81.4	6.22
2017	UCL	9251	766	5375	3341	92.3	73.4	87.5	78.0	81.8	76.6	12.6
2018	UCL	10449	2094	4047	2143	83.3	82.9	65.9	77.4	83.1	83.0	0.61

Table 21.4 Summary of key results from the polyp localization task at GIANA 17 and 18 challenges

Year	Team	TP	FP	TN	FN	Prec	Rec	Spec	Acc	F1	F2	MRT
Best teams												
2017	NTNU	9287	2053	4859	3393	81.9	73.2	70.3	72.2	77.3	74.8	**3.8**
2018	MMMIL	**9875**	**1630**	**5078**	**2805**	**85.8**	**77.8**	**75.7**	**77.1**	**81.6**	**79.3**	4.17
Performance evolution												
2017	KM	6267	4204	4596	6413	59.8	49.4	52.2	50.5	54.1	51.2	13.0
2018	KM	9496	4055	3662	3184	70.0	74.9	47.4	64.5	72.4	73.8	4.11
2017	ODS_AI - MIT	8657	1676	5279	4023	83.7	68.2	75.9	70.9	75.2	70.9	37.3
2018	$ODS\_AI - MIT$	9637	1344	5312	3043	87.7	76.0	79.8	77.3	81.4	78.1	18.89
2017	LIP6	3650	11355	2375	9030	24.3	28.8	17.3	22.8	26.4	27.7	73.3
2018	LIP6	2403	12579	2218	10277	16.0	18.9	14.9	16.8	17.3	18.3	191.65
2017	NTNU	9287	2053	4859	3393	81.9	73.2	70.3	72.2	77.3	74.8	3.8
2018	NTNU	9478	1345	5281	3202	87.6	74.7	79.7	76.4	80.6	77.0	6.39
2017	UCL	8502	2226	5375	4178	79.2	67.0	70.7	68.4	72.6	69.2	13.4
2018	UCL	9288	3255	4047	3392	74.0	73.2	55.4	66.7	73.6	73.4	2.00

Chapter 22
Polyp Segmentation in Colonoscopy Images

Jorge Bernal and Arnau Real

22.1 Polyp Segmentation SD

We show in Table 22.1 the results obtained by the different teams when dealing with the segmentation of SD images. Several conclusions can be extracted from the analysis of this table. First of all, there is a clear winner in the 2017 edition (CVML) but, in the 2018 edition, teams were closer (probably to the huge increase in segmentation networks appeared within this year). Second, for all cases, DICE scores were higher than Jaccard ones but in the same order, that is, the team that won in DICE also won with respect to Jaccard score. This highlights that both metrics, though complementary, are not enough to solve potential draws between teams and methodologies. We show in this chapter the performance of the different teams that took part of the GIANA 17 and 18 poly segmentation tasks.

We can also observe that standard deviation is around 22% in year 2017 but it is a little higher in the following year. This is accompanied by a general improvement in the overall performance, being the highest mean DICE and Jaccard scores around three points higher in 2018 than in year 2017. Though, in general, all teams showed a consistent performance across the different images in the dataset, some of them were particularly challenging for all the teams. We show an example of these images in Fig. 22.1.

By analyzing these images we can clearly see that segmentation methods have difficulties in those examples where the polyp can hardly be seen (images in the top left or bottom right) or when the whole endoluminal scene is crowded with elements (fecal content in the case of top right, along with a very small polyp), including those that appear as result of poor patient preparation.

J. Bernal (✉) · A. Real
Computer Vision Center and Computer Science Department, Universitat Autònoma de Barcelona, Bellaterra (Cerdanyola del Vallès), 08193 Barcelona, Spain
e-mail: Jorge.Bernal@uab.cat

J. Bernal and A. Histace (eds.), *Computer-Aided Analysis of Gastrointestinal Videos*,
https://doi.org/10.1007/978-3-030-64340-9_22

Table 22.1 Polyp segmentation results. Total number of images: 612 SD images

Team	Mean Jaccard	Std Jaccard	Mean DICE	Std DICE
GIANA 2017				
CVML	**0.72**	0.22	**0.81**	**0.21**
UCL	0.61	0.24	0.72	0.25
SFU	0.67	0.25	0.77	0.22
NII	0.27	**0.21**	0.39	0.25
ODS_AI - MIT	0.47	0.35	0.54	0.38
GIANA 2018				
CVML	0.750	0.219	0.835	**0.185**
FanVoyage	0.716	0.239	0.804	0.226
KM	0.704	0.260	0.790	0.245
MIRC	0.603	0.291	0.702	0.282
ModuLabs	0.481	0.254	0.605	0.265
ODS_AI – MIT	0.622	0.239	0.730	0.250
NTNU	0.670	0.322	0.741	0.324
TencentAI	**0.760**	**0.218**	**0.841**	0.190
Neuromation	0.729	0.254	0.808	0.241
Reutlingen	0.311	0.252	0.419	0.293
SRV UCL	0.744	0.267	0.815	0.254
Winterfell	0.562	0.278	0.672	0.272

22.2 Polyp Segmentation HD

The analysis of polyp segmentation results, shown in Table 22.2, indicates that some of the trends that were observed for the case of SD images are kept for high-definition ones. Again, unit values for DICE scores are higher than Jaccard ones. We also observe an overall improvement in the results between the two editions, being the best team in 2017 (CVML) outperformed in around 10 points by the best one in 2018 (OUS).

As we did for SD images, we show in Fig. 22.2 some examples of those images that were particularly challenging for the majority of the teams, aiming at detecting common elements that could lead to conclusions on why these methods fail on them. We can observe how the different methods have difficulties when locating very small polyps or those lateral ones in which the full contour cannot be observed (or, if it can be seen such as in the bottom right image, it is very diffuse).

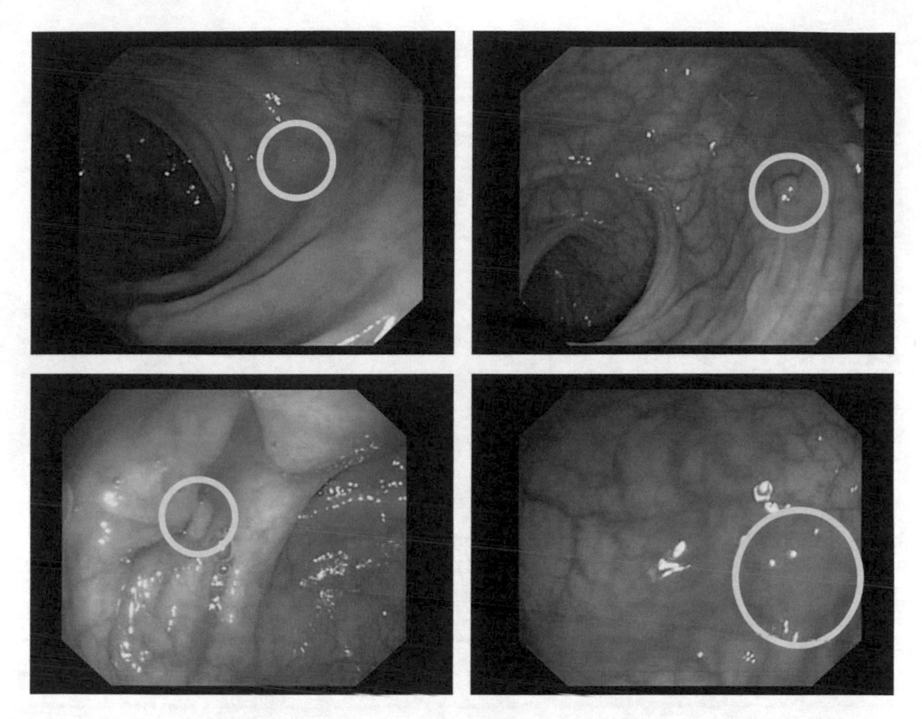

Fig. 22.1 Example of some of the most challenging images for all teams regarding segmentation of SD images. Polyp regions are highlighted by a circle

22.3 Evolution of Results

As we did for the analysis of polyp detection and localization results, we show in Tables 22.3 and 22.4 a summary of the most relevant results extracted by observing carefully the previously presented tables.

With respect to SD images, the winning team in the 2018 edition (PenguinAI) outperformed the winner of 2017 (CVML) in both Jaccard and DICE metrics by a margin of a 3%. We can also observe how all teams clearly improved their game between editions, especially for the case of ODS_AI and $SRVUCL$ which improved their scores by more than a 10%.

The analysis of HD images yields very similar results. Again there was a change with respect to the winning team, CVML in 2017 and PenguinAI in 2018. Differences between the performance of the best teams were higher than in the case of SD images, showing differences close to a 10% in both DICE and Jaccard scores. Contrary to what happened with SD images, not all the teams that took part in both editions showed an improvement regarding the segmentation of HD images; CVML showed a slight improvement whereas SRV UCL really outperformed themselves but, surprisingly, ODS_AI lowered their performance by a small margin.

Table 22.2 Polyp segmentation results. Total number of images: 150 HD images

Team	Mean Jaccard	Std Jaccard	Mean DICE	Std DICE
GIANA 2017				
CVML	**0.74**	**0.20**	**0.83**	**0.18**
UCL	0.40	0.27	0.52	0.28
SFU	0.70	0.24	0.80	0.20
ODS_AI - MIT	0.64	0.28	0.73	0.28
GIANA 2018				
CVML	0.756	0.190	0.844	0.159
FanVoyage	0.683	0.264	0.774	0.247
KM	0.755	0.203	0.841	0.172
MIRC	0.718	0.263	0.799	0.247
$ODS\_AI - MIT$	0.572	0.219	0.699	0.208
NTNU	**0.872**	**0.145**	**0.923**	0.120
TencentAI	0.801	0.203	0.869	0.182
Neuromation	0.740	0.265	0.814	0.249
SRV UCL	0.802	0.241	0.861	0.227
Winterfell	0.508	0.291	0.618	0.294
XMU	0.841	0.157	0.904	**0.112**

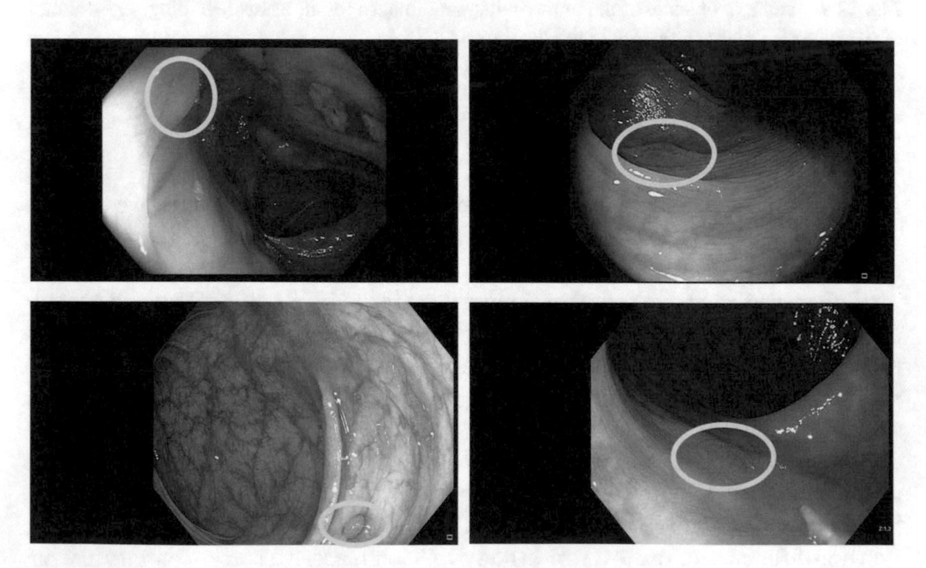

Fig. 22.2 Example of some of the most challenging images for all teams regarding segmentation of HD images. Polyp regions are highlighted by a circle

Table 22.3 Summary of the most relevant polyp segmentation results in SD images over the two editions of the GIANA challenge. Total number of images: 612 SD images

Year	Team	Mean Jaccard	Std Jaccard	Mean DICE	Std DICE
Best team					
2017	CVML	0.72	0.22	0.81	0.21
2018	PenguinAI	**0.760**	**0.218**	**0.841**	**0.190**
Performance evolution					
CVML	2017	0.72	0.22	0.81	0.21
CVML	2018	0.750	0.219	0.835	0.185
UCL	2017	0.61	0.24	0.72	0.25
SRV UCL	2018	0.744	0.267	0.815	0.254
ODS_AI - MIT	2017	0.47	0.35	0.54	0.38
$ODS\_AI - MIT$	0.622	0.239	0.730	0.250	

Table 22.4 Summary of the most relevant polyp segmentation results in HD images over the two editions of the GIANA challenge. Total number of images: 150 HD images

Year	Team	Mean Jaccard	Std Jaccard	Mean DICE	Std DICE
Best team					
2017	CVML	0.74	0.20	0.83	0.18
2018	NTNU	0.872	0.145	0.923	0.120
Performance evolution					
CVML	2017	0.72	0.22	0.81	0.21
CVML	2018	0.756	0.190	0.844	0.159
UCL	2017	0.40	0.27	0.52	0.28
SRV UCL	2018	0.802	0.241	0.861	0.227
ODS_AI - MIT	2017	0.64	0.28	0.73	0.28
$ODS\_AI - MIT$	0.572	0.219	0.699	0.208	

Chapter 23
Wireless Capsule Endoscopy Image Analysis

Aymeric Histace

23.1 Introduction

As explained in previous chapters, in 2017 and 2018, an evolution of the tasks of GIANA challenge related to WCE was proposed. More precisely, in 2017, it was the first time that a task focusing on lesion detection for WCE was proposed in the context of an international challenge, and a particular focus was done on vascular lesions detection. Consequently, the classification/detection task was indeed binary with, on one hand, normal images from WCE presenting with no type of lesions, and, on the other hand, an equivalent subset of images mainly presenting angiodysplasia.

The proposed task was challenging but we clearly saw that it could be improved in terms of difficulty level so it was decided in 2018 to propose a multiclass classification/detection tasks by including a new category to manage: inflammatory lesions that could be seen as more challenging to define and delineate, even for physicians.

As a consequence, the results are presented accordingly to the metrics introduced specifically for each of the year of the challenge.

23.2 2017: Angiodysplasia Detection and Localization

Table 23.1 shows results of angiodysplasia lesion detection and localization.

As it can be noticed in Table 23.1, global performance for angiodysplasia detection and localization is very good both at the sensitivity and specificity levels.

All participating teams for the detection task not only obtained very high performance in terms of precision with a min at 96.9% and a max at 100% but also in terms of specificity. A very interesting point here is that it is not really possible to make a

A. Histace (✉)
ENSEA, ETIS UMR 8051 (CY Paris Cergy University, ENSEA, CNRS),
6 av. du Ponceau, Cergy, France
e-mail: aymeric.histace@ensea.fr

J. Bernal and A. Histace (eds.), *Computer-Aided Analysis of Gastrointestinal Videos*,
https://doi.org/10.1007/978-3-030-64340-9_23

Table 23.1 WCE angiodysplasia detection and localization results

Team	TP	FP	TN	FN	Prec	Rec	Spec	Acc	F1	F2
Lesion detection										
KM	297	6	294	3	98.0	99.0	98.0	98.5	98.5	98.8
ODS.ai - MIT	294	0	300	6	100.0	98.0	100.0	99.0	98.9	98.4
PG	297	6	294	3	98.0	99.0	98.0	98.5	98.5	98.8
NTNU	299	1	299	1	99.7	99.7	99.7	99.7	99.7	99.7
SRV UCL	278	0	300	22	100.0	92.7	100.0	96.3	96.2	94.0
TU/e-VCA	292	1	299	8	99.6	97.3	99.7	98.5	98.5	97.8
UMinho	283	9	291	17	96.9	94.3	97.0	95.6	95.6	94.8
Lesion localization										
KM	295	15	288	30	95.1	90.7	95.0	92.8	92.9	91.6
ODS.ai - MIT	305	4	300	20	98.7	93.8	98.7	96.2	96.2	94.8
PG	296	9	294	29	97.0	91.1	97.0	93.9	93.9	92.2
NTNU	306	8	299	19	97.4	94.1	97.4	95.7	95.7	94.8
SRV UCL	272	17	300	53	94.1	83.7	94.6	89.1	88.6	85.6
TU/e-VCA	302	7	299	23	97.7	92.9	97.7	95.2	95.2	93.8
UMinho	287	187	291	38	60.5	88.3	60.8	71.9	71.8	80.9

strong separation between deep-learning-based methods and more classic one using colorimetric approaches (UMinho). This is probably due to the fact that for this first challenge, very typical vascular lesions were considered with a strong contrast on the mucosa and a very typical saturated red color. It is important to emphasize here that these kind of lesions are the ones that are highly targeted by physicians as they are the most likely to be related to micro-bleeding. It is then very interesting to see that even ad hoc methods, compared with deep learning ones, can provide very high performance.

Looking at the results of localization, we can notice that a gap appears between ad hoc and machine-learning-based methods as a result of the task being more challenging since a bounding box has to be given as an output. Though the ad hoc approach of UMinho remains competitive, the precision falls to 60.5% whereas for other approaches this performance indicator remains high with a mean value around 97.0%. The same can be noticed for the specificity metric, which logically leads to a strong difference when considering F1 score. This can be explained by the fact that the ad hoc method here, based on colorimetric analysis for part of the algorithm, is more sensitive to illumination and can lead to an overestimation of the area depending on the position of the WCE cam with respect to the lesions.

Nevertheless, it is very interesting to emphasize that even ad hoc methods can lead to very good results in detection as they are not demanding in computational resources and that they can handle the task without a strong need for a huge amount of annotated data which still is a primary challenge in the clinical field, including WCE.

As a conclusion here, it is important to highlight that this first attempt to propose detection/localization tasks on WCE in the context of GIANA challenge was a real success and showed the potential of deep-learning-based methods to address typical vascular lesion detection/localization. It was also a good opportunity to show that ad hoc methods are not totally out of the race and thus can lead to very satisfying results when the detection task is considered, without the need of huge computational resources. It could then be imagined that ad hoc color-based method can be a first low-cost filter for fast detection and very complementary to deep-based approaches.

It also appeared that it was important to increase the difficulty level of the tasks for a next challenge on this particular topic in order to push proposed approaches to their limits. A way to address such an objective was to consider more challenging lesions, which means vascular lesions of different types, but also new types of lesions considered as of primary importance by physicians and that also brought a higher level of difficulty because of their clinical characteristics.

23.3 2018: Multilabel Detection and Localization

For the 2018 challenge, following the conclusions of previous challenge, a third category of images was added to the tasks, and inflammatory lesions became part of the detection/localization challenge. These types of lesions are quite interesting since they can take very different forms from one to another. At a very early evolution level, they can be confused with angiodysplasia, when evolving to next steps, ulceration can appear, showing a yellow/white area inside the inflammatory part and making it fully different.

To increase even more the difficulty of the tasks, we also decided to slightly change the content of the vascular lesion database by adding less typical angiodysplasia that, as just said, can be sometimes confused with inflammatory lesion at a very early stage.

As explained in related chapters about database and metrics, adding this new category of inflammatory lesions leads us to propose different kind of metrics for evaluation, extracted from the classic confusion matrix.

Table 23.2 shows results of WCE lesion detection.

Table 23.3 shows results of WCE lesion localization.

Considering lesion detection task (Table 23.2), compared with 2017 challenge, one can notice that the objective of increasing the level of difficulty was fulfilled: we have a more important variety with respect to performance of each participating team, and more than that, having a quick look to TU/e-VCA team, who took part in the 2017 challenge with very high performance, one can notice that the overall accuracy decreased to 88.4% by adding a new category. Another strong difference is the fact that all methods proposed are based on deep learning approaches and that no ad hoc methods took part in the challenge.

On the overall, the mean class accuracy for each team is very satisfying as, if we exclude the worst performance (46.4%), we obtained a minimum value of 87.7%. Surprisingly, at the detection level, the challenge did not come finally from the

Table 23.2 WCE lesion detection results

Team	Global Acc	NIA	IIA	VIA	MeanClassAcc
Lesion detection					
FanVoyage	93.5	96.7	94.4	95.7	95.6
KM	95.5	99.8	95.7	95.5	97.0
$ODS.ai - MIT$	36.6	46.0	47.1	46.1	46.4
TencentAI	94.3	99.7	94.4	94.5	96.2
SRV UCL	88.7	91.6	91.7	93.2	92.1
TU/e-VCA	88.4	98.3	89.1	89.1	92.1
UB	82.6	89.6	86.5	87.0	87.7

Table 23.3 WCE lesion localization results

Team	TP	FP	FN	Prec	Rec	F1	F2
Inflammatory lesions							
FanVoyage	493	247	112	66.6	81.5	73.3	78.0
KM	471	75	134	86.2	77.8	81.8	79.4
$ODS.ai - MIT$	434	221	171	66.2	71.7	68.9	70.6
TencentAI	456	477	149	48.8	75.4	59.3	68.0
SRV UCL	430	327	175	56.8	71.0	63.1	67.7
Yimei	356	27566	249	1.3	58.8	2.5	5.9
Vascular lesions							
FanVoyage	432	155	170	73.6	71.7	72.7	72.1
KM	564	20	38	96.6	93.7	95.1	94.2
$ODS.ai - MIT$	562	106	40	84.1	93.4	88.5	91.3
TencentAI	558	81	44	87.3	92.7	89.9	91.6
SRV UCL	523	98	79	84.2	86.9	85.5	86.3
Yimei	554	28830	48	1.9	92.0	3.7	8.7

inflammatory lesion by their own, but by the fact that we also add some "confusing" vascular lesions in the angiodysplasia database. This can be appreciated by looking at the related performance in the IIA (Inflammatory) and VIA (Vascular) columns where the performance remains quite homogeneous.

It also appears that the identification of normal images was a quite easy task since two teams reaches more than 99% in the specific category. This may lead to an overestimation of the global accuracy and probably could lead to another strategy for future challenges which can be proposed to mitigate this effect.

At the localization level, it is quite interesting to see that the challenging aspect of the tasks appears fully achieved considering the obtained performance. In terms of precision and recall, the best team (KM) obtained a 86.2%, 77.8% for inflammatory lesions and a 96.6%, 93.7% for vascular lesions. Two things can be said here: first of all, the localization tasks strongly discriminate here with a clear advantage for vascular lesions in terms of easiness. All of the teams, except one, managed to obtain (very) satisfying results on this category whereas for inflammatory lesions, the variability is definitely more important starting at 48.8%, 75.4% (excluding the team with the worst obtained results) to 86.2%, 77.8% for the best one, with intermediate teams at 66.0%, 71.7%. It shows that the fact that inflammatory lesions can have very different aspects depending on the evolution stage can lead to a strong dependence to the deep architecture used. It is also linked to the fact that semantic segmentation architectures are less easy to tune and can depend strongly on the way the learning stage is parameterized (loss function, batch, etc.). This is also illustrated by the fact that one team has very poor results although using a classic architecture that has already shown good performance for other kind of applications.

The very interesting point here is the fact that there is room for improvement considering the multilabel tasks. If, in 2017, one could argue that the detection/localization of angiodysplasia could be considered as a solved task on typical vascular lesion due to the very high performance obtained by deep learning approaches, the 2018 datasets brought new challenges and improvement is still possible to have a clear impact on the computer-assisted reading of WCE data.

Chapter 24
Conclusions and Perspectives

Jorge Bernal and Aymeric Histace

The objective of this book was to present several methodologies that have been proposed during the last few years aiming to assist clinicians in some of the most demanding gastrointestinal endoscopy tasks. More precisely, we focus on the analysis of those methods targeting polyp characterization (detection and segmentation) in colonoscopy images and wireless capsule endoscopy lesion detection and localization.

It is clear that, by a simple analysis of the different methodologies proposed, deep learning approaches suppose today the state of the art for all the studied tasks, clearly outperforming classical hand-crafted ones due to their higher capability to generalize from examples. This difference is bigger for the case of colonoscopy video analysis as the large number of images available for sure helps the network to learn polyp appearance with more reliability.

We close the book with this chapter in which we make a brief summary of the main findings that we have observed by the analysis of the different experiments that were carried out during the different challenges, as well as proposing future lines in which validation frameworks could be improved to reflect, even more faithfully, the performance of a given method. We break down this chapter into the two types of images that have been analyzed throughout the book.

J. Bernal (✉)
Computer Vision Center and Computer Science Department, Universitat Autónoma de Barcelona, 08193, Bellaterra (Cerdanyola del Vallès), Barcelona, Spain
e-mail: Jorge.Bernal@uab.cat

A. Histace
ENSEA, ETIS UMR 8051 (CY Paris Cergy University, ENSEA, CNRS), 6 av. du Ponceau, Cergy, France
e-mail: aymeric.histace@ensea.fr

J. Bernal and A. Histace (eds.), *Computer-Aided Analysis of Gastrointestinal Videos*,
https://doi.org/10.1007/978-3-030-64340-9_24

24.1 Colonoscopy Image Analysis

The analysis of colonoscopy images by means of artificial intelligence can be considered already a mature research field. More than 20 years with new developments almost each month makes it a research domain in which innovation is difficult to achieve. With the advent of deep learning networks, differences between methodologies are way smaller than they were in the early 20s where hand-crafted methods were popular. Due to the high popularity of some of the public datasets that are used in this challenge, polyp detection has been the task that has attracted more attention during both GIANA 2017 and 2018.

When GIANA 2017 was proposed, there was no fully publicly available annotated dataset containing videos for the case of colonoscopy image analysis, and $CVC\_VideoClinicDB$ appeared as the first and largest one in the research domain. Though it is weakly labeled (providing ellipses as ground truth instead of pixel-wise masks) the length and variability of the videos soon made it the one to use to train and validate the different methodologies. It has to be mentioned that, to preserve the fairness in the results, ground truth for the testing images was never made public; we offered participants an online evaluation tool in which they could test their methods in a subset of test videos. This initiative was greatly appreciated by the different teams, allowing them to propose improvements to their methodologies up until the last minute.

The analysis of the results achieved by the different methods clearly indicate that it is the time to advance to the next level and test these methods in real procedures. Just to make ourselves clear, the videos from our datasets are indeed from real patients, but the way images are acquired do not represent exactly the way a clinician would manage in a real-life scenario. Those that helped us to build our datasets paid special attention to capture each and every one of the different views of the polyps that appeared in the sequences, which was particularly useful to train the different methods. We plan to incorporate the analysis of full procedures in future iterations of the challenge, provided that we find a way to efficiently annotate large video sequences.

Proposed methodologies are already able to accurately detect and locate all the different polyps that appear in the videos under a reasonable computation time. There is still work to be done in the spatio-temporal coherence of the outputs provided by the methods as the majority of them treat each frame individually, therefore not considering outputs provided before when dealing with a new instance. Besides, the majority of the methods focus on the characterization of the polyp as the ground from which to build up their methodologies, forgetting about the rest of the elements that could also assist on polyp detection/localization such as specular highlights or folds.

Polyp segmentation has not yet achieved the level of attention than polyp detection and localization have. There can be several reasons behind this being the main one that, in fact, there is no clear clinical target behind it. It is true that polyp segmentation can be seen as an intermediate step for polyp classification in a way such the content of the polyp region is deeply analyzed to determine lesion histology but it is also true that many of the available object detection networks do already provide a class for each detected object. Second, the number of polyp segmentation databases (and, more particularly, their size) is very limited: the majority of the available ones contain very few samples, many of them grouped around a same polyp thus presenting a reduced variability in global polyp appearance. This makes it difficult to train and validate a deep learning network from scratch and leads to the use of fine-tuning to efficiently train the network. We have introduced in this book the first publicly available dataset of HD images, which will be enlarged soon and complemented with polyp histology to allow its use for both polyp segmentation and classifications tasks.

Segmenting the region that the polyp occupies in the image could also be useful to assist clinicians in lesion removal or, when used in polyp classification ones, to assist on in vivo histology prediction using lesion size as a cue. Nevertheless, it is clear that this task is not yet mature and that more effort should be made on proposing datasets and also on defining new meaningful metrics, as we have observed how Jaccard and DICE are not particularly complementary with respect to the performance of a given method.

24.2 WCE Image Analysis

It is interesting to see that from 2017 to 2018 the tasks related to WCE attracted much attention with a significant amount of participating teams (7 in 2017, and a total of 8 in 2018). It is quite an important point since WCE is becoming a very strong alternative to classic endoscopy making small bowel examination easier compared with enteroscopy from instance.

Inflammatory lesion, coupled with vascular lesion of different types, is a very challenging task that shows real ambition for future improvement. It would have been very interesting in 2018 to have at least one participant with an ad hoc approach in order to have a common point with 2017: if deep learning method and above all semantic segmentation approaches obtained the best performance on every type of images and lesions, they are still very demanding in terms of computational resources. Ad hoc approaches beyond the simple aspect of performance can bring insight on the explainability of the considered features and could help to have a better understanding of the psychovisual mechanism used by physicians. Bridging this with deep learning architecture would certainly be of great interest as it is not that easy right now to have a good understanding of the underlying mechanisms of some architecture nor the reliability one can have on the results even if good from a quantitative point of view (considering standard metrics).

Another topic of interest for next challenges on WCE is, of course, to propose a bigger annotated database, even if it remains a real challenge considering the fact that annotation is a really high time-consuming task for clinicians, especially at the segmentation level. This latter is, however, necessary if we want to address semantic segmentation task that could lead finally also to characterization of the lesions, which remains an open challenge.

Lesion characterization could be considered from two perspectives: first, at the level of providing quantitative parameters on the lesion (size, area, perimeter, compacity, etc.) that can be related to clinical features and then help the physician to categorize the type of lesions among a particular type, and even more challenging to consider the pertinence level of a lesion which needs to take into account during the learning process a new type of information making it even more interesting. Nevertheless, for the latter, it also means to have access to new databases proposing this kind of data, and only a few initiatives have been started since 2019 (CAD-CAP database in one of the few) and time will be needed to propose a significant and reliable set of images.

A last challenge for future iterations of GIANA will be to consider several types of video capsules. Until now, the CAD-CAP database used for the challenge has focused only on the main constructor on the market, leading more than 95% of the selling, Medtronics and the Pillcam (SB3). Several alternatives can be considered right now including Olympus, Ankon, or OMOM. Image characteristics can be slightly different depending on the sensor used for image acquisition and it could have influence on the performance related to lesion detection/localization which have to be estimated for a same kind of pathology. Again, we are facing the curse of database here, and time is needed to gather significant amount of data with reliable annotations.

Methodologically speaking, finally, it would be very interesting to propose a task related to data and ground truth computer-assisted generation as it has been proposed in other fields of applications. GAN, few-shot learning, variational encoder approaches can be seen as core strategy to strengthen competitivity of the approaches regarding the small amount of data with respect to classic challenges in computer vision/machine learning communities.

24.3 Overall Conclusions

Gastrointestinal image analysis, as it has been shown in this book, is a clearly active research topic. This is proven by the amount of new publications appearing daily and with the increasing interest of manufacturers on including artificial intelligence modules as part of their devices. This book has shown how different methodologies can be used to tackle a same problem and that some of them already present a performance level that could warrantee their use in a clinical scenario.

It is clear that these systems should be tested under real-life conditions to complete their validation but still the variability of the different datasets that we have used for the experiments should be seen as a proof of concept of the performance of these methods in the exploration room.

The objectives of this book were both to introduce to the general and specialized public the work that has been done in the field of gastrointestinal image analysis as well as to present a validation framework that can be used for any given method to test its performance. It is clear that more tasks could have been explored and deeper analysis could have been provided but we do believe that this book really shows what we pretended at the beginning of its writing: gastrointestinal image analysis is here to stay and to assist clinicians in a meaningful way. Thank you very much for accompanying us in this first book; hopefully, there will be more to come in the future with new tasks, methods, and analysis.